Bodybuilding Supplements

The Ultimate Guide to Bodybuilding Diets

(Gain Strength and Muscle Size With Nutrition Secrets)

Leona Walker

Published By **Elena Holly**

Leona Walker

Bodybuilding Supplements: The Ultimate Guide to Bodybuilding Diets (Gain Strength and Muscle Size With Nutrition Secrets)

ISBN   978-1-77485-961-2

No part of this guidebook shall be reproduced in any form without permission in writing from the publisher except in the case of brief quotations embodied in critical articles or reviews.

Legal & Disclaimer

The information contained in this ebook is not designed to replace or take the place of any form of medicine or professional medical advice. The information in this ebook has been provided for educational & entertainment purposes only.

The information contained in this book has been compiled from sources deemed reliable, and it is accurate to the best of the Author's knowledge; however, the Author cannot guarantee its accuracy and validity and cannot be held liable for any errors or omissions. Changes are periodically made to this book. You must consult your doctor or get professional medical advice before using any of the

TABLE OF CONTENTS

Chapter 1: My Aching Joints And Cod Liver Oil

Thank God for Youtube! I had serious knee pain going up stairs. When I went for an x-ray, it showed that I did not have arthritic knees. The knee specialist prescribed physical therapy and to stop climbing stairs. I already trained my legs at least once a week so I didn't see how more exercise was going to help them. I was a mover and going up stairs is part of the job. I wasn't about to quit, so I turned to Youtube.

I found a video about cod liver oil and joint pain. Apparently, <u>a study had been done</u> where patients who had been on pain medication, received 1.5 grams of cod liver oil per day and reported a significant decrease in pain.

Well, crap, that was enough for me. I ordered some Cod Liver Oil. I took 2000 mg every day. Now, i kid you not---my knee pain completely disappeared within a week! I am not exaggerating. You mean simply taking Cod Liver Oil eliminated my joint pain? YES! I couldn't believe it either. No offense to doctors (well maybe some) but no doctor, no physical therapist, no joint specialist, and no x-ray tech suggested this to me. I got this from YOUTUBE!

I was pleased at the results, but also annoyed that none of these practitioners could turn me on to this when there were studies that show that Cod Liver Oil works!

What is Cod Liver Oil and how does it work?

Cod liver oil is a nutritional supplement derived from the liver of cod fish. As with most fish oils, it has high levels of the omega-3 fatty acids, eicosapentaenoic acid (EPA), and docosahexaenoic acid (DHA). Cod liver oil also contains high levels of vitamin A and vitamin D. It has historically been taken because of its vitamin content. It was once commonly given to children, because vitamin D has been shown to prevent rickets--whatever that is. Google it.

Vitamin A is a strong antioxidant (meaning it can prevent cell damage in your body by interacting with harmful molecules called free radicals which are produced within the cells). Vitamin D plays an important part in the production of proteoglycan in cartilage as well as helping to maintain a healthy musculoskeletal system.

Cod liver oil was traditionally manufactured by filling a wooden barrel with fresh cod livers and seawater, and allowing the mixture to ferment for up to a year before removing the oil. Modern cod liver oil is made by cooking the whole cod body tissues of fatty fish during the manufacture of fish meal.

The two types of omega-3 fatty acids found in fish oil are DHA and EPA. These can reduce inflammation, which causes swelling and pain. Together, these factors can make fish oil a potential weapon against arthritis. The EPA and DHA found in cod liver oils attack the enzymes that cause inflammation in the joints.

EPA and DHA can also help prevent heart attacks by making it harder for the blood to clot. They help lower blood triglyceride levels and blood pressure, too.

They significantly reduce the release of several elements that play a part in inflammation from your white blood cells.

They, also, form the building blocks for prostaglandins, which regulate your immune system and fight joint inflammation. Omega-3 fatty acids also play a role in lowering cholesterol and triglyceride levels in your blood, so they can reduce the risk of heart disease and stroke in people with inflammatory arthritis.

Other Fish oils higher in EPA and DHA might work as well. A precaution here is not to take too much in order to avoid Vitamin A overdosing which is bad for the liver. I have been taking 2000 mg of Cod Liver every morning for years and it has completely alleviated my joint pain. Every man should be taking fish oils, in my humble but accurate opinion.

Chapter 2: Garlic For Cardiovascular Health

With my success in dealing with my joint pain, I began to ask: are there other conditions that I have that could be treated by nutrition and exercise that the medical community was not making known to me?

One of my issues was borderline high blood pressure, or hypertension. Hypertension runs in my family and both my grandfather and uncle died from stroke.

As I described in the introduction, when I was diagnosed with mild hypertension, the first thing my doctor did was prescribe a medication called Lisinopril.

This medication caused me to get a bad rash. It took me a long time and a biopsy to discover that Lisinopril was the culprit. I was convinced I had bed bugs or dust mites, or some other horror. No, it was the Lisinopril. I immediately stopped taking it and again sought out some natural aides. I did some research on blood pressure.

Every time you get your blood pressure checked, you get two numbers. These numbers tell you how hard your blood pushes against the walls of your arteries as it flows through your body. The higher figure, called systolic pressure, indicates the force pushing on blood vessels as the heart contracts. The lower figure, called diastolic pressure, shows the force when the heart relaxes.

A healthy blood pressure reading is below 120/80. There's no single cutoff between healthy and unhealthy numbers, but most doctors agree that -- among people up to 59 -- a blood pressure reading above 140/90 is high blood pressure; in people 60 and over, a reading of 150/90 calls for medical management. In these ranges, both the heart and arteries are straining too hard to move blood. This condition is called hypertension or high blood pressure, and it affects about one in three U.S. Adults. Two things that affect your blood pressure greatly is obesity and salt intake.

OBESITY

Even a small loss of weight can lead to a reduction in blood pressure. Though this is not a weight loss book (coming soon) it's amazing that even a small reduction in belly fat can have a significant effect on your blood pressure.

In a new study at the American Heart Association's <u>High Blood Pressure Researcher 2014 Scientific Sessions</u>, scientists from the Mayo Clinic in Rochester, Minnesota, reported that blood pressure increase was specifically related to weight gain around the abdominals, called belly fat.

Blood pressure rises with body weight, so losing weight is one of the best ways to improve your numbers. According to the national guidelines and recent research, losing weight can lower both systolic and diastolic blood pressure -- and potentially eliminate high blood pressure. For every 20 pounds you lose, you can drop systolic pressure 5-20 points. People who are considered pre-hypertensive can benefit significantly by dropping 20 pounds. In my fitness book, coming soon, I discuss that the simple fact is that calorie control is the key factor in weight loss, not exercise alone. Suffice to say, I undertook a physical regime which included calorie restriction and exercise. This helped greatly.

SALT

Americans eat more salt and other forms of sodium than they need. Often, when people with high blood pressure cut back on salt, their blood pressure falls. Cutting back on salt also prevents blood pressure from rising. So cutting back on calories and salt will help lower your blood pressure, and so will exercise. But there is also a supplement that helps lower blood pressure and it is garlic!

GARLIC

<u>In Recent randomized controlled trials</u> that compared garlic to placebo in patients with hypertension, it appears that garlic may have some blood pressure lowering effect. Please

click on the links so you can see the studies for yourself.

Garlic is an herb. It is best known as a flavoring for food. But over the years, garlic has been used as a medicine to prevent or treat a wide range of diseases and conditions. The fresh clove, or supplements made from the clove, is used for medicine.

Garlic is used for many conditions related to the heart and blood system. These conditions include high blood pressure, high cholesterol, coronary heart disease, heart attack, and "hardening of the arteries" (atherosclerosis). Some of these uses are supported by science. Garlic actually may be effective in slowing the development of atherosclerosis and seems to be able to modestly reduce blood pressure.

The chief agent in Garlic is allicin. Allicin has been found to have numerous antimicrobial properties. Allicin has antiviral activity both in vitro and in vivo. Among the viruses susceptible to allicin are Herpes simplex type 1 and 2, Parainfluenza virus type 3, human

Cytomegalovirus, Influenza B, Vaccinia virus, Vesicular stomatitis virus, and Human rhinovirus type 2.

Allicin works to decrease blood pressure chiefly through vasodilation. Vasodilation refers to the widening of blood vessels. It results from relaxation of smooth muscle cells within the vessel walls, in particular in the large veins, large arteries, and smaller arterioles. In essence, the process is the opposite of vasoconstriction, which is the narrowing of blood vessels. It has an interesting chemical effect in the body to achieve this.

The Studies:

Garlic has been proven to lower Blood Pressure! Click the links for read the following studies.

Garlic supplementation prevents oxidative DNA damage in essential hypertension

Aged garlic extract lowers blood pressure in patients with treated but uncontrolled hypertension: a randomised controlled trial

Lipid-lowering effects of time-released garlic powder tablets in double-blinded placebo-controlled randomized study.

According to the research, which you can link to and read for yourself, Garlic has definitive properties that LOWER BLOOD PRESSURE!

Meanwhile, no doctor told me any of this. I was put on Lisinopril which gave me a serious allergic reaction. Not only that but....

GARLIC HAS BEEN PROVEN TO LOWER LDL (BAD) CHOLESTOEROL!

More Studies:

Garlic as a lipid lowering agent--a meta-analysis.

Effect of garlic on serum lipids: an updated meta-analysis.

Garlic's is a powerful anti oxidant that may help with aging, dementia, and alzeiheimers.

I don't know about you, but these studies are enough to convince me that Garlic supplementation is a good idea. While many prefer to consume garlic as food, the way my diet works it is better for me to use supplementation.

I found when I stopped taking the garlic my systolic pressure crept up 10 points.

Chapter 3: Penis Envy - L Citrulline And Nitric Oxide

Let's face it, as men age, the quality of their erections degenerate. That really sucks. This is a complaint that I had when I went to my doctor. His immediate reaction was to suggest Cialis and Viagra! But what is the underlying problem? Is there a way to deal with the issue without dangerous pharmaceuticals?

That's what I wanted to find out. As I did some research, I discovered that one of the key factors in an erection is Nitric Oxide!

Nitric Oxide is a very important chemical in your body-- NOT TO BE CONFUSED WITH NITROUS OXIDE or laughing gas. Nitric oxide was discovered to be a neurotransmitter in the nerve cells that control erections. Are you still interested?

In addition, in mammals, including humans, Nitric Oxide is an important cellular signaling molecule involved in many physiological and pathological processes._It is a powerful vasodilator with a short half-life of a few seconds in the blood. That means it helps blood flow everywhere in your body. EVERYWHERE! By dilating (expanding) the arteries, nitric oxide drugs lower arterial pressure and left ventricular filling pressure. Long-known pharmaceuticals such as nitroglycerine and amyl nitrite were found to be precursors to nitric oxide more than a century after their first use in medicine.

There have been over 60,000 studies done on nitric oxide in the last 20 years and in 1998, The Nobel Prize for Medicine was given to three scientists that discovered the signaling role of nitric oxide.

How does Nitric Oxide Work?

The interior surface (endothelium) of your arteries produces nitric oxide. When plaque builds up in your arteries, called atherosclerosis, you reduce your capacity to produce nitric oxide, which is why physicians prescribe nitroglycerin for heart and stroke patients. Also, age, and hypertension will decrease nitric oxide levels.

Another way to increase nitric oxide is through diet, most notably by consuming the amino acids L-arginine and L-Citrulline. Arginine can be found in nuts, fruits, meats, and dairy, and directly creates nitric oxide and citrulline inside the cell.

L-Citrulline is a substance called a non-essential amino acid. Your kidneys change L-Citrulline into another amino acid called L-Arginine and consequently, nitric oxide. Taking L-Citrulline may be better than taking L-Arginine directly because L-Arginine loses much potency in the digestive tract. L-Citrulline seems to be more efficient in producing nitric oxide in the body. Some advocate taking both L-Citrulline and L-Arginine together. These compounds are important to your heart and blood vessel health. They may also boost your immune system.

When L-Citrulline enters the kidney, vascular endothelium and other tissues, it can be readily converted to Arginine, thus raising plasma and tissue levels of Arginine and enhancing nitric oxide production.

Increasing nitric oxide has become the new secret weapon for athletes and bodybuilders. Athletes are now taking supplements with L-Arginine and L-Citrulline to support the flow of blood and oxygen to the skeletal muscle. They also use them to facilitate the removal of exercise-induced lactic acid build-up which reduces fatigue and recovery time.

Since Arginine levels become depleted during exercise, the entire Arginine-Nitric oxide-Citrulline loop can lose efficiency, causing less-than-ideal nitric oxide levels and higher lactate levels. Supplements can help restore this loop allowing for better workouts and faster recovery from workouts.

Supplementation with L-Citrulline may increase the body's production of nitric oxide more effectively than L-Arginine, because much L-Arginine consumed directly is lost in the digestive process. L-Citrulline avoids intestinal or liver metabolism and enters the kidneys, where it is rapidly converted into L-Arginine. Since L-Arginine is much less active in the kidneys, the majority of the L-Arginine produced there from L-Citrulline is not siphoned off, but goes back into the circulation and is thus made available to the vascular and penile endothelium.

Nitric Oxide affects many organs. It helps as a neurotransmitter in the brain. It helps to dilate blood vessels and has a calming effect.

The Studies:

Oral L-citrulline supplementation improves erection hardness in men with mild erectile dysfunction.

Enhanced Exercise Tolerance

Research on the body's usage of L-Citrulline during exercise suggests that consuming a citrulline supplement might enhance performance. A study published in 2011 in the

"Journal of Nutritional Science and Vitaminology" reported that laboratory animals fed L-Citrulline and subjected to intense exercise were able to perform longer and also had lower levels of blood ammonia and lactate, two waste compounds produced during exercise, than a placebo group.

Another study published in the March 2012 issue of the "International Journal of Cardiology" found that healthy male subjects who consumed L-Citrulline for seven days had improved arterial function because arterial walls were less stiff, compared to a placebo group. These are positive findings, but both studies were small, and larger clinical trials are still needed to confirm Citrulline's cardiovascular benefit.

Citrulline deals with the CAUSE of Erectile Dysfunction, Viagra Doesnt.

I take 3 grams of Citrulline morning and night. I take the powdered form in water. It has SIGNIFICANTLY improved my erections and I believe has also helped to lower blood pressure. I would not go a day without it.

Get Inexpensive Citrulline Supplements Here!

Chapter 4: Vitamin D

Vitamin D was also something I was lacking in my annual blood test. Many men are lacking in this key vitamin. Sometimes it is due to our not getting enough sunlight, but why is Vitamin D important? Vitamin D is a fat-soluble vitamin that is naturally present in very few foods, added to others, and available as a dietary supplement. It is also produced when ultraviolet rays from sunlight strike the skin and trigger vitamin D synthesis.

Vitamin D promotes calcium absorption in the gut. It is also needed for bone growth and bone remodeling by osteoblasts and osteoclasts. Without sufficient vitamin D, bones can become thin, brittle, or misshapen. Vitamin D prevents rickets in children and osteomalacia in adults. Rickets again... Okay here. Together with calcium, vitamin D also helps protect older adults from osteoporosis.

There are some groups of people that are more likely to have vitamin D deficiency. The following people are more likely to be lacking in vitamin D:

People with darker skin. The darker your skin, the more sun you need to get the same amount of vitamin D as a fair-skinned person. For this reason, if you're Black, you're much more likely to have vitamin D deficiency than someone who is White.

People who spend a lot of time indoors during the day. For example, if you're housebound, work nights, or are in hospital for a long time.

People who cover their skin all of the time. For example, if you wear sunscreen or if your skin is covered with clothes.

People that live in the North of the United States or Canada. This is because there are fewer hours of overhead sunlight the further away you are from the equator.

Older people have thinner skin than younger people and this may mean that they can't produce as much vitamin D.

Infants that are breastfed and aren't given a vitamin D supplement. If you're feeding your baby on breast milk alone, and you don't give your baby a vitamin D supplement or take a supplement yourself, your baby is more likely to be deficient in vitamin D.

People who are very overweight (obese). Scientists speculate that it might be because Vitamin D is sequestered in fat, or becomes too diffused throughout the body.

Worldwide, an estimated 1 billion people have inadequate levels of vitamin D in their blood, and deficiencies can be found in all ethnicities and age groups. Indeed, in industrialized countries, doctors are even seeing the resurgence of rickets, the bone-weakening disease that had been largely eradicated through vitamin D fortification.

Why are these widespread vitamin D deficiencies of such great concern? Because research conducted over the past decade suggests that vitamin D plays a much broader disease-fighting role than once thought.

Being "D-ficient" may increase the risk of a host of chronic diseases, such as osteoporosis, heart disease, some cancers, and multiple sclerosis, as well as infectious diseases such as tuberculosis and even the seasonal flu.

The Studies:

<u>Several studies link low vitamin D levels with an increased risk of fractures in older adults</u>, and they suggest that vitamin D supplementation may prevent such fractures—as long as it is taken in a high enough dose.

Vitamin D and Multiple Sclerosis: Multiple sclerosis (MS) rates are much higher far north (or far south) of the equator than in sunnier climes, and researchers suspect that chronic vitamin D deficiencies may be one reason why. One prospective study to look at this question found that among white men and women, those with the highest vitamin D blood levels had a 62 percent lower risk of developing MS than those with the lowest vitamin D levels.

<u>A promising report in the Archives of Internal Medicine</u> suggests that taking vitamin D supplements may even reduce overall mortality rates: A combined analysis of multiple studies found that taking modest levels of vitamin D supplements was associated with a statistically significant 7 percent reduction in mortality from **any cause**.

Vitamin D supplementation seems to be a good idea not just for men but for everyone. I take 2000 I.U. every morning and every evening and have gotten the "OK", from the doctor that I am no longer "D-ficient"

Chapter 5: Saw Palmetto And The Prostate

When urinating I was finding that occasionally my stream was not what it should be and I was having a dribbling effect afterwards. Why does nature become our enemy after 50? Good grief! I knew that this probably meant I was developing BPH, yet my doctor told me my prostate was normal.

BPH, also known as benign prostatic hyperplasia, is a benign increase in the size of the prostate gland. An estimated 50% of men have evidence of BPH by age 50 and 75% by age 80; in 40–50% of these men, BPH becomes clinically significant.

The prostate gland is a walnut sized gland near the bladder. Unfortunately, the increase in size of this gland can lead to problems, like difficulty in urination because the prostate puts pressure on the urethra as it enlarges.

BPH is a pain. It causes you to get up during the night to urinate. It makes you feel you have to go more often.

What Causes BPH?

Doctors are not exactly sure what causes benign prostatic hyperplasia. The changes that occur with male sex hormones as part of the aging process seem to play a role in the enlargement of the prostate gland.

Male hormones affect prostate growth. The most important male hormone is testosterone, which is produced in the testes throughout a man's lifetime. The prostate converts testosterone to another powerful androgen, dihydrotestosterone (DHT).

DHT stimulates cell growth in the tissue that lines the prostate gland (the glandular epithelium) and is the major cause of the rapid prostate enlargement that occurs between puberty and young adulthood. DHT is a prime suspect in prostate enlargement in later adulthood.

The female hormone, estrogen, may also play a role in BPH. (Some estrogen is always present in men.) As men age, testosterone levels drop, and the proportion of estrogen increases, possibly triggering prostate growth.

So if DHT, (which is a product of the prostate metabolizing testosterone) causes the prostate to grow, then how do you stop this process?

One method is castration. No testicles, no testosterone, means no DHT. I doubt many want to go this route.

Rather than eliminating testosterone, which we all want for male potency, we want to limit the DHT. This is where Saw Palmetto comes in.

What Is Saw Palmetto?

Saw Palmetto extract is an extract of the fruit of Serenoa repens. It is rich in fatty acids and phytosterols. It has been used in traditional, eclectic, and alternative medicine to treat a variety of conditions, most notably benign prostatic hyperplasia (BPH).

The Saw Palmetto plant produces small berries that contain several natural compounds with biological activity. These include a group of fatty compounds called plant sterols, such as beta-sitosterol, campesterol, and stigmasterol. These compounds have anti-inflammatory activity, according to experts at Memorial Sloan-Kettering Cancer Center, and may also block the activity of a cellular enzyme called 5-alpha reductase. This enzyme converts the main male sex hormone, testosterone, into its metabolite, DHT. Although the cause of BPH is not totally understood, excess production of DHT in the gland is probably involved. Saw Palmetto compounds may reduce the amount of DHT available to prostate cells by as much as 40 percent, according to Sloan-Kettering experts.

Some research suggests that saw palmetto compounds may be helpful in controlling DHT production in men who already have BPH.In one clinical study published in the May 2000 issue of "Urology," researchers measured DHT levels in prostatic biopsy specimens from men with BPH who took either a saw palmetto supplement or a placebo for six months. They found that DHT levels were reduced by 32 percent in the group taking saw palmetto, compared to the placebo group.

Saw palmetto is used in several forms of traditional herbal medicine. American Indians used the fruit for food and to treat a variety of urinary and reproductive system problems. The Mayans drank it as a tonic, and the Seminoles used the berries as an expectorant and antiseptic.

More Studies:

Improving BPH symptoms with Saw Palmetto NCBI

Research seemed to indicate that the extract brought about a "mild to moderate improvement in urinary symptoms and flow measures."

Since taking Saw Palmetto, I found my urinary symptoms improving and so far my Dr. has found no prostate enlargement. So I will be keeping it up. I take 275mg of Saw Palmetto in the morning and evening.

Chapter 6: Stinging Nettle

There is another herb that I found that helps with BPH issues. Another herb touted as relieving some of the symptoms of BPH is Stinging Nettle Root. I was beginning to have some bathroom issues, needing to go frequently, etc. When I started taking the Stinging Nettle, I found those trips to the bathroom lessening. While taking Stinging Nettle, I maybe have to go once during the night. Sometimes I last the whole night without going. Stinging Nettle (Urtica dioica and the closely related Urtica urens) has a long medicinal history. In medieval Europe, it was used as a diuretic (to rid the body of excess water) and to treat joint pain.

Stinging Nettle has fine hairs on the leaves and stems that contain irritating chemicals, which are released when the plant comes in contact with the skin. The hairs, or spines, of the Stinging Nettle are normally very painful to the touch. When they come into contact with a painful area of the body, however, they can actually decrease the original pain. Scientists think nettle does this by reducing levels of inflammatory chemicals in the body, and by interfering with the way the body transmits pain signals.

Stinging Nettle has been used for hundreds of years to treat painful muscles and joints, eczema, arthritis, gout, and anemia. Today, many people use it to treat urinary problems during the early stages of an enlarged prostate (called benign prostatic hyperplasia, or BPH). It is also used for urinary tract infections, hay fever (allergic rhinitis), or in compresses or creams for treating joint pain, sprains and strains, tendonitis, and insect bites.

Benign Prostatic Hyperplasia (BPH)

Stinging Nettle root is used widely in Europe to treat BPH. Studies in people suggest that Stinging Nettle, in combination with other herbs (especially Saw Palmetto), may be effective at relieving symptoms such as reduced urinary flow, incomplete emptying of the bladder, post urination dripping, and the constant urge to urinate. These symptoms are caused by the enlarged prostate gland pressing on the urethra (the tube that empties urine from the bladder).

Some studies suggest that Stinging Nettle is comparable to finasteride (a medication commonly prescribed for BPH) in slowing the growth of certain prostate cells. However, unlike finasteride, the herb does not decrease prostate size. Scientists aren't sure why nettle root reduces symptoms. It may be because it contains chemicals that affect hormones (including testosterone and estrogen), or because it acts directly on prostate cells. It is important to work with a doctor to treat BPH, and to make sure you have a proper diagnosis to rule out prostate cancer.

Osteoarthritis

The leaves and stems of nettle have been used historically to treat arthritis and relieve sore muscles. Some small studies suggest that some people find relief from joint pain by applying nettle leaf topically to the painful area. Other studies show that taking an oral extract of Stinging Nettle, along with nonsteroidal anti-inflammatory drugs (NSAIDs), allowed people to reduce their NSAID dose.

Hay fever

One preliminary human study suggested that nettle capsules helped reduce sneezing and itching in people with hay fever. In another study, 57% of patients rated nettles as effective in relieving allergies, and 48% said that nettles were more effective than allergy medications they had used previously. Researchers think that may be due to nettle's ability to reduce the amount of histamine the body produces in response to an allergen. More studies are needed to confirm nettle's antihistamine properties. Some doctors recommend taking a freeze-dried preparation of Stinging Nettle well before hay fever season starts.

Other

Preliminary animal studies indicate that nettle may lower blood sugar and blood pressure. However, more research is needed to determine whether this is also true in humans.

More Studies:

The inhibiting effects of Urtica dioica root extracts on experimentally induced prostatic hyperplasia in the mouse.

Urtica dioica for treatment of benign prostatic hyperplasia: a prospective, randomized, double-blind, placebo-controlled, crossover study.

These studies suggest that Stinging Nettle Root is effective in relieving some of the symptoms of BPH.

I can tell you from experience that taking Stinging Nettle Root in the morning and evening has significantly reduced middle of night urination. I take one 500mg capsule every morning and evening.

Chapter 7: Milk Thistle And Your Liver

Another result of my age 50 medical checkup was that I was diagnosed with Fatty Liver. I don't consider myself an alcoholic but I was a pretty liberal drinker, until the doctor told me that I had fatty liver. Let's get real, by the time you are 50, your liver has lived a little and processed a lot of alcohol and other things. Your liver is the chief filter for your body.

Some fat in your liver is normal, but if it makes up more than 5%-10% of the organ's weight, you may have fatty liver disease.

There are two main types of fatty liver disease:

• Alcoholic liver disease (ALD)

• Nonalcoholic fatty liver disease (NAFLD)

Alcoholic Liver Disease (ALD)

You can get alcoholic liver disease from drinking lots of alcohol. It can even show up after a short period of heavy drinking. Genes that are passed down from your parents may also play a role in ALD. They can affect the chances that you become an alcoholic, and they can also have an impact on the way your body breaks down the alcohol you drink.

Other things that may affect your chance of getting ALD are:

• Hepatitis C (which can lead to inflammation in your liver)

• Too much iron in your body

• Being obese

Nonalcoholic Fatty Liver Disease (NAFLD)

It's not clear what causes this type of fatty liver disease. It tends to run in families. It's also more likely to happen to those who are middle-aged and overweight, or obese. People like that often have high cholesterol and diabetes as well.

Other causes are:

- Medications

- Viral hepatitis

- Autoimmune or inherited liver disease

- Fast weight loss

Diagnosis of Fatty Liver Disease

You might find out that you have the disease when you get a routine checkup. Your doctor might notice that your liver is a little larger than usual.

Other ways your doctor might spot the disease are:

Blood tests. A high number of certain enzymes could mean you've got fatty liver.

Ultrasound. It uses sound waves to get a picture of your liver.

Biopsy. After numbing the area, your doctor puts a needle through your skin and takes out a tiny piece of liver. He looks at it under a microscope for signs of fat, inflammation, and damaged liver cells.

In my case, it was discovered through an ultrasound test. The danger of this disease is that it can progress into Cirrhosis, which is a scarring of the liver and that can lead to other complications. Treatment involves reducing the risk factors, such as obesity, through a diet and exercise program. It is generally a benign condition, but in a minority of patients, it can progress to liver failure (cirrhosis).

The other wise thing is to limit or avoid alcohol since it can only exacerbate the condition. If it is due to Hepatitis, then there are vaccines like the Hepatitis B vaccine, Hepatitis A vaccine but there is also a supplement I found that has a beneficial effect on the liver.

Milk Thistle is an herbal supplement that detoxifies and protects vital liver functions and more. Milk Thistle has been used for over 2,000 years as a natural treatment for liver disorders. The plant is known in scientific circles as the Silybum marianum, but it is more commonly known as "milk thistle," "St. Mary Thistle," "Holy Thistle," and "Lady's Thistle." It is an herbaceous annual or biennial plant belonging to the Asteraceae family that can grow to be 10 feet tall with flowers that are red and purple in color.

Milk Thistle seeds contain a bioflavonoid complex known as Silymarin. Silymarin, which is the active ingredient in milk thistle, is simply the purified extract of the fruits (seeds) of the milk thistle plant. It is responsible for the main medical benefits of the milk thistle plant, and it is made up of three main flavonoids:

silybin – also known as silibinin

silydianin – also known as silidianin

silychristin – also known as silicristin

Double blind studies on the effect of milk thistle on toxic liver damage (mostly alcohol-related), chronic liver disease, and disease caused by certain drugs have been reviewed by medical experts.

The Studies:

MILK THISTLE IN LIVER DISEASE PAST, PRESENT AND FUTURE

A REVIEW OF PLANTS USED IN THE TREATMENT OF LIVER DISEASE

The experts all concluded that Milk Thistle is an extremely therapeutically useful medicinal plant product that stabilizes the cell membrane and stimulates protein synthesis while accelerating the process of regeneration in damaged liver tissue. These effects are important in the therapeutic efficacy of milk thistle.

According to other studies, Milk Thistle may protect the cells of the liver by blocking the entrance of harmful toxins and helping remove these toxins from liver cells. As with other flavonoids, Milk Thistle is a powerful antioxidant which works to maintain health and energy by protecting the body from

43

damage caused by free radicals and lipid peroxidation, which can injure healthy cells and tissues.

Of course, if you have any serious liver disease, you should consider your alcohol intake and the recommendations of your doctor. Be kind to your liver, it's the only one you got!

I take 250mg morning and evening, My doctor tells me I still have fatty liver and it could be diet related, so he told me to consume less fat, (not so many bacon, egg and cheese sandwiches!) and drink more water.

Chapter 8: The One Medication I Take - Clomiphene

DISCLAIMER: This drug is not currently FDA approved for men, but women only.

With this disclaimer out of the way, let me show you why Clomiphene is one of the best medications you can take for hormone therapy. As I told you in my introduction, when I came from my checkup, the doctor told me that my free testosterone was about 150 ng/dl (nanograms per deciliter) which is quite low. I figured as much because of the symptoms I was experiencing of low libido and weak performance.

The urologist that I was referred to actually did steer me away from testosterone patches and creams because of the dangerous side effects. All he could recommend to me was to take a pre testosterone hormone called DHEA. That helped a little, but really wasn't cutting it. So it was back to the internet.

Before I describe what I found let's examine the issue of low testosterone:

Whether you are a 30, 50, 80, or even 110 year old man, having low testosterone levels (hypogonadism) is neither fun nor healthy. The symptoms of low testosterone in men range from lack of energy, depressed mood, loss of vitality, muscle atrophy, muscles aches, low libido, erectile dysfunction, and weight gain...to bone loss, osteoporosis, mild anemia, increased risk of Alzheimer's, increased risk of high-grade prostate cancer, and increased risk of death due to all causes.

As you may know, low testosterone in men may be caused by problems in the testes (or gonads). This is called <u>primary hypogonadism</u> and can be brought on by the mumps, testicular trauma, or testicular cancer, etc., and can only be treated with testosterone replacement therapy. **However, the more common causes of low testosterone/hypogonadism result from problems in the pituitary gland and/or hypothalamus in a man's brain.** Low testosterone levels caused by such "brain problems" are collectively described as <u>secondary hypogonadism</u> or hypogonadotropic hypogonadism and may result from depression/anxiety, head trauma, iron overload, anabolic steroid overdosing, diabetes, sleep deprivation, or some medications.

Traditionally, if low testosterone is diagnosed, testosterone replacement therapy is prescribed, and it most commonly comes in the form of a cream, gel, pellet, patch, and by injection. Although these types of therapy are effective, some methods are better than others, and there are side-effects with all of them.

For example, testicular shrinkage, gynecomastia (breast enlargement), low sperm count/sterility, and polycythemia (overproduction of red blood cells) are common side-effects of testosterone replacement therapy (for many sufferers, these side-effects are mostly treatable or considered "worth it" by the patient).

But I found something that causes the body to produce more of its own testoterone!

Clomiphene Citrate

However, specifically due to the sterility side-effect, such testosterone treatments aren't a good option for men who want to have children. In these (usually young) hypogonadal men, clomiphene citrate (CC pill, or Clomid), and/or human chorionic gonadotropin (HCG) have been used (by specialists) for decades to increase testosterone production, increase sperm production, and increase fertility.

Both these therapies effectively help signal the testes to produce testosterone and thereby increase testosterone levels (assuming of course the cause of the initial problem is not in the testes' ability to make testosterone).

My doctor and a specialist recommended DHEA, Cialis and Viagra, or testosterone replacement therapy for my Low Testosterone. But after exploring the internet again -- what an incredible thing -- I found out about Clomiphene, otherwise known as Clomid. It turns out that Clomid is a drug prescribed often to <u>women</u> with fertility issues.

Let me try to explain how it works. In a healthy male, the pituitary gland in the brain releases luteinizing hormone (LH) into the blood stream, which signals the testes to "GO" and produce testosterone.

Pituitary produces LH-----Signals "Go" Testes----Testes Produce Testosterone----Testosterone converts to Estrogen---Estrogen signals Pituitary "Stop producing LH".

After testosterone has been produced it naturally converts to some estrogen (yes, there's estrogen in men, too) and this estrogen acts as a "STOP" signal to the pituitary to stop making LH.

Clomiphene also "tricks" the hypothalamus to produce more releasing hormone (GnHR), which in turn travels to the pituitary gland to increase LH and FSH production. LH and FSH in turn increase testosterone production, and sperm production, thus maintaining and enhancing fertility.

Clomid (clomiphene citrate) works by blocking estrogen at the pituitary and hypothalamus. Thus, the usual estrogen message to "STOP" production of LH is essentially silenced, and therefore the pituitary makes more LH and there is an increased "GO" signal to produce testosterone in the testes. HCG works by mimicking LH, which also increases the "GO" signal to produce more testosterone in the testes.

The best thing about Clomid is that it stimulates the body to produce its own testosterone, whereas testosterone introduced from the outside, actually signals the testes to shut down because THE BODY THINKS IT HAS ENOUGH AND MORE testosterone is not needed!

Again, clomiphene is not FDA approved for men. Why is that? Could it be that big pharmaceutical companies are against it, because it is a cheaper and more effective alternative to their Low Testosterone therapies? Just saying.

I began taking 25mg tablets of Clomid on a daily basis. It turned on my own natural testosterone machine and my levels went from 156 nl into the 600's! This had a profound effect on my life.

Chapter 9: Building Your Foundation

Eating for Muscle and Strength

Supplements have the capacity to give your body the enhanced fuel that it needs to get bigger and stronger than you thought possible without resorting to illegal drugs. They can also help you to strip fat from your body and super charge your energy reserves. But supplements are just that - supplements. They are supplementary to sound nutrition and training regimens. Unless you get your eating plan and your workout programs on point, all of your supplementary investments will one big waste of cash. Here, then, are the key principles upon which your mass and strength training nutritional program should be based:

Eat every 3 waking hours

Make breakfast your biggest meal of the day, taking in about 20% of your total daily calories

To gain mass, consume 500 calories more than your daily maintenance level of calories

Consume 1 gram of protein per pound of body weight

Eat a balanced mix of macronutrients in the following ratio: 55% Carbs / 30% Proteins / 15% Fats

Focus on lean protein sources such as salmon, flounder, skinless chicken, egg whites and lean red meat

Get a mix of starchy and fibrous carbs at each meal

Drink 2.5 liters of water each day

Have a meal one hour before and about 45 minutes after your workout

Ensure that you are getting essential fatty acids in your diet, especially Omega-3 Fatty Acids.

Nutrient Timing

Breakfast, Lunch and Dinner. It's when we eat. Always have done. Why change now?

Well, for one thing, the way that the Western world has been eating over the last hundred or so years hasn't really reaped too much in the way of positive health benefits. In fact, we are sitting slap, bang in the middle of the worst obesity epidemic in human history. Maybe that's got something to do with the timing of those meals. Let's find out.

The way we eat is contrary to logic. Most people have a pretty light breakfast. Yet, by definition, breakfast comes at the end of a 12 to 16 hour fast. At the start of the day our bodies crave energy. We need to get a decent meal into our systems. By lunchtime most people are hanging out for some nutrition and end up having a hearty lunch. But then at night, when they're planning to do little more than sit in front of the TV and go to sleep they take in a huge amount of food. This inverted pyramid model - not much in the morning, a medium amount at lunch and a heap in the evening - is part of the reason that so many of us are losing the battle against fat. We need a better plan.

The human body works most efficiently when it is supplied with a constant supply of energy. The smart way to supply it is to eat every three waking hours. Eating 3 meals a day will not allow you to achieve your fat loss goals. Strange as it may sound, you have to eat more often than that in order to lose the weight. In fact, you should be eating every 3 waking hours. Obviously your meal portions will be much smaller than the traditional 3 meals per day. Each meal will have the same calorie count. The macronutrient ratio will also be the same (except for your post exercise meal, which will have a little more protein). Here are 5 reasons why eating every 3 hours is the smart way to go:

It provides a regular, ongoing energy supply throughout the day, meaning that you'll feel more energetic all day long.

It helps to stop grazing and binging. In fact, you'll have that satisfied, full feeling most of the time. If you do feel like a snack, the fact that your next scheduled meal is not far away will help you to curb the urge.

You will more efficiently absorb protein. Your body can only absorb 30 grams of protein at any one time. Large meals often exceed that amount and that means that a portion of that much needed protein is wasted. Smaller, regular portions will overcome this problem.

It boosts the metabolism. The very act of eating burns calories. So, the more you eat, the more calories you'll be burning. As long as what you're eating is healthy and your calories are regulated, that's got to be a good thing.

It is psychologically healthy: Rather than depriving yourself of food, it is far better psychologically to eat more regular but smaller meals. Doing so helps you to view food as your body's fuel source, which is exactly what it is.

Ideal meal size

Your ideal meal size will depend upon your total daily calorie requirements. Once you have established this number, simply divide it by the number of meals that you are eating each day. So, if you are taking in 2,400 calories per day and are eating 6 meals per day, then you'll be taking in 400 calories per meal. That's probably less than half of what you're eating for dinner at the moment.

100 Nutrition Tips

Before you even think about spending money on supplements you simply have to get your foundational eating plan on point. Here are 100 nutritional tips that you'll want to nail before going to the next level with supplements

To control your party eating, have a healthy meal before you go, such as a bowl of soup or a slice of whole grain bread.

Maintain a fruit bowl on the kitchen table that is stocked with washed fresh fruit daily. Have apples, pears and bananas ready to eat. If they spoil get rid of them quickly.

Whether making granola or cooking something else, use canola oil. Of all oils, it's lowest in artery-clogging saturated fat.

Cut and bag vegetables or prepare other snacks ahead of time. Then, you can just reach in the refrigerator for a quick and portable snack.

Muffins can be great sources of fiber. Forget the restaurant variety and make low fat muffins at home that are high in fiber.

The darker green the lettuce you choose, the more nutrients it contains. Deep green, yellow, orange and red vegetables pack vital vitamins.

Frozen fruit makes smoothies easy. Just combine low-fat or fat-free milk and a cup of frozen berries and blend. Add a little honey if the berries aren't sweet enough.

The snacks in most vending machines are loaded with salt and sugar. Avoid them at all costs.

Salad bars can provide plenty of healthy options. However, watch out for the fatty foods such as salad dressings and cheese.

Most restaurants serve large portions. Divide a meal in half and share it or take it home for another meal.

Chicken skin contains most of the fat in chicken. Skinless chicken, especially white meat, is a great low-fat choice. It pays to take the effort to remove that skin.

Fast foods are not always junk foods. They can be nutritious. Many fast food meals include a meat sandwich, french fries and soda. This combination provides complex carbs and protein. Just don't overdo it.

Most people who eat a well balanced diet don't need vitamin supplements. Food is a better source of vitamins and minerals than supplements - it not only has the right balance of nutrients but also many other healthy substances.

Fruit juice is a healthier choice than soda because it contains many needed vitamins.

For a healthier alternative to soda, combine 240 mls of fruit juice with 120 mls of carbonated water.

The most common allergy producing fruits and vegetables are apples, peaches, strawberries, tomatoes, potatoes, celery, onions, parsley and citrus fruits.

To help prevent disease eat two pieces of fruit and 5 servings of vegetables a day. That equates to about one and a half cups of vegetables per day.

Health bars, such as muesli or yoghurt bars are often high in sugar and fats. They are usually not very healthy at all!

Most nutrients in fruits and vegetables are maintained when you choose frozen, canned or fresh varieties. Cooking can reduce nutrients so steam quickly to preserve them.

Add some fresh spinach leaves to salads for extra fiber, vitamins, minerals, anti- oxidants and flavor.

Eat a range of fruits and vegetables to get a bigger variety of important nutrients. One example is the phytochemicals in citrus fruit.

Fruits are high in sugars such as sucrose and fructose. These sugars are easily absorbed and burn in the body as carbohydrate energy. Soluble fiber in fruit slows the absorption of these sugars, meaning that you get healthy, sustained energy.

Foods such as eggs can have different names on food labels. Look out for albumen, apovitellin, avidin, flovoproteins, livetin, lysozyme, ovalbumin and powdered egg.

The most common ingredients causing food reactions are shellfish, eggs, fish, milk, nuts and sesame seeds.

Look out for 'Omega-3" symbols on food labels for milk, margarine, eggs and cans of tuna. Use the symbol to help you to get your essential fatty acids.

A takeaway burger, large fries and drink contains about 1000 calories. A healthier choice is a ham, cheese and salad multigrain roll, with just 400 calories.

Getting enough protein is easy. Cereal and milk for breakfast equals 10 grams of protein. A typical steak will give you 30 grams. And a single egg equates to 13 grams of protein.

People need to eat a variety of protein foods for amino acids. Eating a variety of proteins gives us the essential amino acids we need for healthy bones, skin, hair and nails.

Foods such as eggs, fish and dairy products are high in biological protein. The protein in these foods comes with other healthy nutrients, giving your body a nutrient boost.

Solid waste from the body, called faeces, tells us if we are eating well. Healthy faeces are soft and bulky.

Soya beans differ from other beans because they have more fat. But it is a polyunsaturated fat that is good for you.

Levels of heart disease are very low in countries around the Mediterranean Sea. They eat a very healthy diet containing lots of fruit and vegetables, little fish, lean meat, olive oil and a small amount of wine.

Smoking increases the need for Vitamin C. Smokers should increase their daily intake of Vitamin C by drinking an extra glass of fresh orange juice each day.

Milk and milk products prevent your teeth from holes and decay. This is because dairy food can reduce acidity in your mouth, stimulate saliva and reduce plaque formation.

Most dairy foods are excellent sources of calcium. Other foods that contain calcium are fish with edible bones, almonds, brazil nuts, sesame seeds, dried fruit and dark- green, leafy vegetables.

For naturally good health, eat low-fat calcium fortified dairy foods such as milk on calcium fortified cereal or a slice of low-fat cheese on a multi-grain bread sandwich.

Low-fat dairy, as part of a healthy diet, may help prevent bowel cancer and diabetes. it may even have a role in maintaining healthy weight.

Water is the best thing you can drink when you are thirsty. However, a milk drink is better than soft drink or cordial.

Calcium and zinc are need in the chemical reaction that makes energy in the body. They are catalysts during the production of energy from glucose.

Soft cheeses, such as ricotta, do not have much calcium. Do not include them when you count your daily servings of dairy food.

Cow's milk contains nearly all of the important nutrients humans need, including high-quality protein, calcium, vitamin-A, vitamin B-12 and zinc.

Eat some organic fruits and vegetables and compare the flavor with regular fruits and vegetables. Organic growers claim that their food tastes better. What do you think?

Store dry foods such as rice, flour and sugar in sealed containers to keep them fresh and safe from pests.

Buy fresh foods from local markets and support local farmers and gardeners - you'll also be getting the freshest produce available.

When choosing packaged foods, select the ones that have 'no added salt' marked on the packaging.

There are 2 types of fiber, insoluble and soluble. You need both for good health. Insoluble fiber is the hard part of the food, like apple skin. Soluble fiber is in the cells that give foods, such as apples, their shape. Oats, baked beans and lentils are high in soluble fiber.

For good health, you should have 15-25 grams of fiber a day. That could constitute a bowl of high fiber cereal or two pieces of fruit.

Remember to eat your crusts. The crusts on bread contain healthy anti-oxidants.

Bread is a good energy source. It is a low-fat food, rich in complex carbohydrates and fiber. Wholemeal and multigrain breads have more fiber, minerals and vitamins than refined white bread.

Try to choose medium Glycemic Index (GI) foods that are in the 51-69 GI range to get the most efficient sources of energy from your foods.

It is important to eat plant foods, because they contain starch and our body uses starch for energy.

Onions are believed to have a blood cleansing ability. It is a healthy, cheap vegetable which contains lots of nutrients.

Did you know that eating fish or peanut butter sandwiches can help you get better test scores? They contain hormones that improve your brain function.

A table spoon of Greek yogurt before every meal helps absorb fat.

Foods that contain too much sugar can cause damage to your teeth, tooth decay and gum disease as well as causing bad breath. If you want fresh breath stay away from sweet things.

Make at least half of your carbohydrate foods whole grain each day.

Keep the skin and peels on fruits and vegetable if possible.

Eat a crispy fresh salad instead of one with oily dressing or mayonnaise.

Dark chocolate contains lots of healthy nutrients. Just don't over-indulge.

Avocado and peanut butter both provide and abundance of healthy fats. Use them liberally.

Fresh lemon juice can be utilized by the liver to produce more enzymes than any other food element.

Ginger has been proven to provide an amazing array of health benefits. It has, in fact, been called a wonder food.

Sea vegetables are an amazing source of nutrients and vitamins. Sprinkle them on any dish to provide a more healthy option.

Want to burn a quick 25 calories? Simple - drink a glass of ice-cold water.

Eating plenty of vegetables helps you get all the vitamins your body needs - we need vitamin A for good eyesight and to fight infection.

Make sure that you eat at least one dark green and one orange vegetable every day.

We need some fats and oils to absorb some vitamins. We also use some fats to grow new nerves.

Yogurt is a great way of protecting your boy against ulcers. It also helps to digest foods better.

Tomatoes, broccoli, red capsicum and oranges are very high in vitamin C.

Cordial, soda and drinks that are high in sugar actually dehydrate the human body.

Vitamin A and D are often added to milk, making milk a very healthy choice to drink instead of soda or any other drinks high in sugar.

Salt is very high in sodium which is why seasoning your food with lots of salt can become a very bad habit that can lead to high blood pressure and heart attack.

Limit yourself one all-purpose multi-vitamin daily.

To add a nutritional boost to pasta sauce, throw in some diced vegetables like eggplant, carrots or spinach.

It is important that you think and find out about what is in your food, then you will be able to make educated healthy choices about what to eat and drink.

For a great source of fiber, omega-3 fatty acids and protein give hemp protein a go.

Persimmons are a great source of fiber and vitamin A. They are also packed full of other essential nutrients.

Want an easy way to grill your steak - grab a George Foreman Grill. It really works!

Strawberries are packed full of nutrients goodness. A serving has more vitamin C than an orange - and all in just 43 calories.

Chocolate is high in fat, even though it tastes good and contains mostly cocoa butter. A third of the cocoa butter is steric acid which is bad for you.

Eat every 3 waking hours. This will allow you to elevate your metabolism and provide a constant flow of energy all day long.

Set aside one day per week to plan for and prepare your meals for the week. Prepare a double batch of your favorites and freeze them for later.

One can of soda contains 10 teaspoons of sugar and the average American adult drinks up to 500 cans of soda per year - that's about 52 pounds of sugar consumed in soft drinks alone.

Drinking lots of water helps flush away systems of waste products and toxins, yet many people go through life dehydrated causing tiredness, low energy and headaches.

Use fresh fruit and vegetables as center pieces at meals. This will encourage diners to make use of them.

Cut heavy cream from your recipes and replace with evaporated skim milk and cornstarch.

Herbal teas are good for you because they will soothe your frazzled nerves and keep you focused.

Replace regular pasta with spaghetti squash. It has only one quarter of the calories. Slice it in half, remove the seeds and cook in the microwave for 7 minutes.

Eating up to two portions a week of fish can give you your requirement of omega3 which is great for your heart health.

Grill, microwave and sauté vegetables with fish for a mouthwatering dish that will be ready in 6 minutes.

Coconut has some wonderful nutritional qualities. It is an excellent source of selenium

Breakfast is the most important meal of the day. Don't miss it or your brain won't be able to work properly.

Most meats are healthy for you but the most healthiest is fish , because it contains more protein and vitamins than other meats.

Growing brains need certain nutrients from food. "Brain foods" include fish, vegetables such as broccoli, cauliflower, egg yolks and milk.

Make coffee an occasional, rather than a daily, drink. It causes nutrient deficiencies!

Eat more nuts and seeds - walnuts, hazelnuts, brazil nuts, macadamias and pistachios.

The fact that you like to eat a variety of foods is your body's way of telling you that it needs many different nutrients-not just one or two.

Don't eat anything with ingredients you can't pronounce.

Avoid fizzy drinks of all kinds - they contain phosphorous which depletes our calcium levels and makes our bodies acidic.

To get maximum digestion of the food you eat, slow down and chew your food thoroughly.

Chapter 10: Supplement Theory

Why Supplement?

The right supplements - taken at the right times - can help propel you to your bodybuilding and strength training goals by doing three things. They can increase your anabolic drive, improve your workload capacity and decrease your recovery time. Individually these factors can make a big difference. Put together they will work synergistically to power you towards your goals. Let's consider them one at a time:

Anabolic Drive

The word 'anabolic' refers to the body's ability to produce more muscle tissue. Anabolic drive involves the natural production of testosterone, growth hormone (GH), insulin-like growth factor-1 (IGF-1), insulin, thyroid, cortisol and other hormones and growth factors involved in muscle growth. For athletes, it refers to the body's ability to increase its anabolic (or muscle producing) response to exercise, nutrition, supplements and other factors.

In the case of supplements, those targeted towards increasing the production of testosterone, growth hormone and insulin, and decreasing cortisol, will result in both anabolic and anti-catabolic effects, thus maximizing the anabolic drive.

Workload Capacity

Endurance or workload capacity involves your ability to maintain high quality training throughout a workout. If your capacity is limited and you don't have the energy, endurance or concentration necessary to train hard from the beginning of your workout to the end, it won't matter how well you manage the other components - nutrition, supplementation and rest. Your diet may be excellent. You may even be training properly six days a week, but if you don't have the overall energy and muscle endurance for a productive workout, you aren't going to experience maximal progress or muscle growth.

Recovery

This involves your ability to recover properly between sets as well as workouts. The goal is to ensure that the body recovers fully from the stimulus of exercise and to reduce the amount of time necessary for it to take place. Recovery is critical to muscle growth. Your body must recuperate from the catabolic process before productive protein synthesis can occur. The sooner you recover from a workout, the sooner your body can begin to respond to it and adapt by adding muscle.

When you don't recover from workouts, you can go into a state of chronic over training. You'll actually begin to lose muscle instead of gaining it. In the gym, you'll find yourself lacking the energy to do further sets at maximum ability. Even if you do manage to get through a workout without losing effort, your body still won't respond with the kind of adaptation you want - more muscle.

Certain supplements can have a strong effect on lowering recovery time and increasing muscle growth. Supplements targeting recovery can also help you handle additional stress in your training. If you want to extend workouts from four to six days a week, supplements can help you accelerate recovery to make those workouts productive. Similarly, if you're training for another sport, in addition to your bodybuilding and strength training endeavors, supplements might just spell the difference between being able to train for both effectively and having the dual training sabotage your progress in both areas.

Anti-catabolism

You can decrease the breakdown of muscle tissue both during and after exercise and thus provide potent anti-catabolic effects in several ways. A lot of substances and methods decrease muscle breakdown and have anti-catabolic effects; for example taking in adequate carbohydrates is known to have a protein sparing effect.

Certain supplements can also create an anti-catabolic effect. Cortisol is a necessary hormone and in plays a significant role in decreasing muscle stiffness and inflammation. Without normal and somewhat elevated cortisol levels, we couldn't even exercise properly - so it wouldn't matter what training, diet, drug or nutritional supplement regimen you followed. Yet, chronically elevated levels of cortisol have a catabolic effect on muscle and decreases the effect of anabolic hormones. Decreasing the amount of cortisol after exercise can provide you with an added anabolic boost by decreasing muscle tissue breakdown and increasing amino-acid influx and utilization by muscle cells. In addition, decreasing catabolism by using appropriate methods and supplements can dramatically increase protein synthesis and muscle mass.

Substances that decrease catabolism can have anabolic effects on muscle. But like growth hormone stimulation, many nutritional supplements can also have anti-catabolic effects. Increasing dietary calories and protein and using branch chain amino acids, glutamine, alanine and other amino acids, Vitamin C, beta-carotene and other anti-oxidant vitamins have been shown to lessen muscle breakdown.

Supplements can also be used to increase insulin, Growth Hormone, IGF-1 and testosterone levels, and decrease cortisol levels and decrease cortisol levels and other anti-catabolic factors at specific times to maximize increases in lean body mass.

Are There Steroids in those Supplements?

Contaminants - anabolic androgenic steroids and other prohibited supplements - can, indeed, find their way into supplements. The largest survey conducted on this issue was from the International Olympic Committee - accredited laboratory in Cologne, Germany. They looked for steroids in 634 supplements and found that a whopping 15% of them contained substances - including nandrolone - that would lead to a failed drug test. Nineteen percent of UK samples were contaminated. In another study, researchers from the Olympic

Analytical Laboratory at the University of California found that some brands of androstenedione are grossly mislabeled and contain the illegal anabolic steroid, testosterone cypionate. Men who took either 100 mg or 30 mg of androstenedione for one week tested positive for 10-norandrosterone, a metabolic by-product of nandrolone. In another report, Swiss researchers found different substances that those declared on the labels, including testosterone, in seven out of 17 pro-hormone supplements - that is 41% of the supplements that were tested!

The following substances may be found in some supplements but are banned by the International Olympic Committee and, thus, may cause a positive drug test:

Ephedrine

Strychnine

Androstenedione

Androstenediol

Dehydroepiandrosterone (DHEA)

19- Norandrostenedione

19-Norandrostenediol

In most countries, there are currently no specific legislation requirements governing the safety of sports supplements. As they are classified as foods, supplements are not subject to the same strict manufacturing, safety, testing or labeling requirements as licensed medicines. This means that there is no guarantee that a supplement lives up to its claims. Generally the legislative requirements covering vitamin and mineral supplements are more stringent. In some countries, manufacturers can only use nutrients and ingredients from a permitted list, and even then within maximum limits. Each ingredient must undergo extensive safety tests before it is allowed on the permitted list and, therefore, into a supplement. Manufacturers must also provide a scientific proof to support a product's claims and ensure that it is clearly labelled.

Avoiding Scams

When it comes to ads for dietary supplements, it pays to keep the old adage "let the buyer beware" at the forefront of your mind. It can be tricky to separate fact from fiction in product advertisements for diet supplements. Several US government agencies and consumer groups monitor ads and make a valiant effort to try and protect consumers from false and misleading claims. Back in 1997, the Federal Trade Commission carried out "Operation Waistline" - investigating misleading and deceptive weight loss claims - which resulted in penalties against seven manufacturers. More recently the FTC's "Operation Cure-All" looked into misleading and fraudulent online ads involving dietary supplements and other medical miracle products.

The agency took action against Enforma Natural Products, makers of "Fat Trapper" and "Exercise in a Bottle." FTC officials objected to Enforma's ads implying their products could help customers lose weight while they slept, even if they ate lots of fattening foods. Even celebrity endorsers didn't get off easy. The FTC's case against Enforma also included actions against Steve Garvey, who acted as a celebrity endorser in the company's infomercials. The FTC obtained a $10 million settlement from the company on behalf of consumers, but still keeps a close eye on Enforma's continuing questionable practices.

The National Advertising Division (NAD) of the Council for Better Business Bureaus, the advertising industry's self-regulatory forum, has also challenged claims made by makers of numerous dietary supplements and weight loss aids. NAD investigators found that many of the companies used questionable testing techniques or could not provide sufficient proof to support their claims.

Misleading - or downright untrue - advertising sometimes victimizes even the celebrities themselves. Paula Abdul successfully battled makers of a weight-loss drink after the company launched an ad campaign falsely attributing the singer's figure to their product.

Under FTC regulations, claims made by a manufacturer regarding the effectiveness of their product must be substantiated by rigorous scientific studies. Also, if ads show cases involving amazing or unusual results, the company must clarify the typical outcome consumers are more likely to obtain. Manufacturers have gotten creative in trying to dance around these advertising regulations. Eagle-eyed viewers will spot tons of tiny print on ads for dietary supplements. For example, during an ad that promises miracle weight loss, a split-second footnote may note "diet and exercise is required."

Despite the best efforts of groups like the FTC and NAD, it's not easy to police an industry that does $12 billion in annual sales, so consumers must use common sense and a good dose of skepticism in evaluating advertising claims.

The FTC warns consumers to be skeptical of rave reviews by celebrities and other paid endorsers. Although legally these endorsers must be bona fide users of the product if they so imply it in the ad, that's frequently not really the case. Consumers should watch for celebrities who seem to be reciting a script without much conviction, or stars who endorse one product this week, despite hawking a competing product last week.

Obviously, consumers should take testimonials from celebrities and other paid spokespeople with a grain of salt, but even those from "regular Joe's" can be suspect. Consider the case of Bobby Aldredge, who recently appeared in ads for Xenadrine EFX, crediting the product for his 56 pound weight loss and offering impressive "before and after" photos as proof. Observant readers may have found Aldridge's story familiar - the year before he submitted a nearly identical set of photos in the Body - for - Life Challenge - only that time he attributed his weight loss to a host of other supplements, including a competing brand's fat burner.

The FTC says misleading ads often use "buzz words" like scientific breakthrough, miraculous cure, exclusive product, secret ingredient or ancient remedy. They may also claim the government, the medical profession or research scientists have conspired to suppress the product. Here are other examples of suspicious claims that should immediately put you on alert:

"Lose 30 Pounds on 30 days"

As a rule, the faster you lose weight, the more likely you are to gain it back. Also, fast weight loss could harm your health. Unless your doctor advises it, don't look for programs that promise rapid weight loss.

"Lose All the Weight You Can For $39.99"

Some weight loss programs have hidden costs. For example, some don't advertise the fact that you must buy their pre-packaged meals that cost more than the program fees. Before you sign up for any weight loss program, ask for all the costs. Get them in writing.

"Lose Weight While You Sleep."

Claims for diet products and programs that promise weight loss without effort are phony.

Lose Weight and Keep It Off For Good."

Be suspicious about products promising long-term or permanent weight loss. To lose weight and keep it off, you must change how you eat and how much you exercise.

"John Doe Lost 48 Pounds in Six Weeks."

Don't be misled by someone else's weight loss claims. Even if the claims are true, someone else's success may have little relation to your own chances of success.

"Scientific Medical - Miracle Breakthrough"

There are no miracle weight loss (or weight gain) products. To lose weight, you have to reduce your intake of calories and increase your physical activity. Be skeptical about exaggerated claims.

When deciding whether a product can measure up to its ads, ask yourself these questions:

Does the endorsement come from an expert with vague or easily obtained credentials? Some products offer testimonials from people referred to simply as "therapists" or "counselors."

Is there a lot of fine print? Scan the ad for disclaimers indicating the endorser is a paid spokesperson, or does not actually use the product in question.

Are the claims verifiable? Ask the company for proof of its "scientific studies", then see if you can verify those claims yourself.

Does the company have a bad history? Do an online search or check the websites of FTC and NAD for a prior history of offenses. These websites also allow consumers to file complaints about suspicious or misleading ads.

The Truth about Before and After Photos

Those before and after pictures that show amazing body transformations as a result of using a certain supplement are certainly enticing. They're also big business, inducing thousands of desperate people to pull out their credit card and help the supplement industry to record profits. The sad truth of the matter is that - just as you may have suspected - many of them as scams. With the advances in photographic manipulation at marketer's disposal today, it's a cinch to create awesome transformations in days. Photoshop, professional lighting, improved posture, body shaving, tanning and flexing of muscles in the after photo make a ton of difference. In addition, unscrupulous marketing companies often pay in shape bodybuilders and other athletes to get out of shape, allowing a film of fat to cover their muscle. They use terrible posture and an unkempt look to produce terrible before photos. The bodybuilder / athlete then undergo a two or three week training program to get back to the shape that they were in before the process started. More than likely, they will never have touched the product that the company paying them uses their pictures to promote.

There are a series of examples floating around the internet of personal trainers who have taken before and after photos that are actually spaced only about an hour apart in order to demonstrate just how easy it is to fool people into thinking that they have transformed their physique. The bottom line is that creating a quality physique takes years of consistently hard work, disciplined nutrition and getting a sufficient amount of recuperation.

Those Fitness Magazine Ads

Magazines exist to sell supplements. That's why they are packed chock full of glossy, multi-color and multi-page advertisements. In fact many of their "advertorials" are hard to distinguish from the actual articles in the magazine. Many of those real articles finish up with product recommendations anyway.

All they have to do is to keep getting the magazines into the hands of the millions of people around the world desperate to pack muscle onto their frame - and they know they'll make a killing.

Of course, the supplement companies who place the ads in the mags also know that they need to keep coming out with new and novel attention grabbing headlines to keep the punters interested. So, they inundate us with all manner of false ideas about what it takes to pack on the muscle mass.

The reality is that you cannot trust what these magazines tout simply because they are produced by people with a vested interest. The money behind the pages comes from the supplement companies.

Pre-Workout Supplementation

Nutrition sets the foundation for your workout. It is the fuel that will power you through your training sessions. Yet, there is a widespread belief out there that you shouldn't eat before you train. That, though, is the biggest mistake you can make in your training preparation - especially if you are intent on building muscle. You simply must provide your muscles with the right environment to operate at their peak.

When to Eat it

The optimal time to eat is 60 - 90 minutes before the workout if you're concentrating on consuming whole foods. Any sooner than that and you may suffer from gastro-intestinal upset while you're training. Planning then, is critical. Give yourself plenty of time to prepare your meal, so that the time you are actually eating, rather than preparing it, it is within that 60 - 90 minute window. Alternately, prepare your meal ahead of time. The food needs to be well and truly into your bloodstream and coursing toward your muscle cells as you walk through the gym door.

What To Eat

Eating fish pre-workout is a great idea. It is one of the fastest digesting proteins, whereas meat, which is a slow digesting protein will take 3-4 hours to get into your bloodstream. White fish, however, will provide a steady stream of amino acids into your bloodstream just in time for when it counts. This will help promote recovery and prevent catabolism. The fish will provide fast digesting protein. You do not want to eat fat prior to your workout. When you are working out you should be spiking your insulin. You can achieve this by sipping on a workout shake while you're training. Insulin is a storage hormone, so when levels are high, any fat floating around in your bloodstream will go straight to your fat stores. You will, however, need to add some quality carbohydrates. Slow release carbs are the way to go here. Fast release carbs will spike your insulin levels, but you don't want this to happen until you are working out. So, leave it until you are in the gym to spike your insulin. Slow release carbs will provide a steady stream of energy to power you through your workout. Brown rice is a great choice here.

Some alternative pre-workout meals are an apple or a banana with some tuna, a protein shake, or a slice of bread with tuna on it (no butter on the bread).

The Protein Shake Meal

If you choose to take your pre-workout meal in the form of a shake rather than whole food, then you should move it closer to the workout - within 30 minutes of training is ideal. You should be looking for a shake that will give you 20 grams of protein and about 30-40 grams of carbohydrate to provide the ideal environment to carry you through your workout, prevent muscle breakdown and encourage muscle recovery and growth. Whey protein powder is the fastest digesting protein that you can consume. The amino acids in whey protein will get into your bloodstream and to your muscles during the workout, when you need them the most. Whey is also a great source of the branch chain amino acids, Leucine, Isoleucine and Valine, which reduce fatigue and increase energy levels during the workout, as well as keeping your testosterone levels high and reducing muscle breakdown after the workout.

A pre-workout shake will supply your protein needs. For carbs, the best thing you can do 30 minutes before the workout is to eat some fruit like an apple or a banana. Carbs from fruit will provide a slow release energy source without interfering with fat burning. Fruit is also a great choice because it provides powerful antioxidants that maximize nitric oxide levels during training. Research has also shown that polyphenols in such fruit as apples not only increases muscle strength and endurance but also enhance fat burning. (1)

No Carbs?

If you are trying to maximize fat loss, you should consider ditching your pre-workout carbs completely. Even though slow carbs will interfere less with fat burning during the workout than fast carbs, the only way to truly maximize fat burning during the workout is to avoid carbs completely.

Ideally your pre and post workout meals should be no more than 3 to 4 hours apart, with a 45 - 60 minute training session sandwiched between them.

Key Facts

Have a meal 60 - 90 minutes before the workout

Focus on fast release proteins and slow release carbs

Take no fat in your pre-workout meal

Take in 20 grams of protein and 30-40 grams of carbs

If you are taking a pre-workout shake have it 30 minutes before the workout

Your pre-workout shake should be whey protein based

Take an apple with your shake

If on a fat cutting diet, ditch the pre-workout carbs

Overcoming Central Nervous System Fatigue

Ever wondered why some days you simply can't train at the intensity you would like? Your diet hasn't changed, yet you can't train as hard and you feel much more fatigued from the same workout that you blasted through only days before. So, what's causing this plummet in performance? Research has shown that your psychological state can actually affect how many motor units are recruited (a motor unit is a motor unit and all of the muscle fibers it innervates. The more you activate, the more muscle fibers are stimulated, making you stronger and more powerful). (2)

Simply put, your state of mind can determine your levels of strength, and you know that your state of mind can be vastly different in a day-to-day basis. In other words, how you feel mentally affects your exercise performance, your levels of fatigue and, ultimately, your progress. To perform at your best, from a neurological standpoint, it is vitally important that you have an optimal amount of what is called central nervous system "arousal." This is when your brain is stimulated to the point of reaching the ideal environment - the "zone" as some call it - for maximal production and minimal fatigue. The key is reaching an optimal state; too little arousal and performance plummets, but having too much arousal can lead to focus and actually worsen performance.

The major players in nervous system arousal, the factors that promote this optimal "zone", are a class of neurotransmitters called catecholamines, namely epinephrine (adrenaline), norepinephrine (noradrenaline) and dopamine. All act as central nervous system stimulants and affect performance both indirectly by stimulating the central nervous system and directly by exerting their effects on muscles. This close relationship between certain nerve cells, neurotransmitters and hormones has brought about what has been dubbed the neuroendocrine system (nerves that produce neurotransmitters that have both neural and hormonal functions).

Exercise is actually one of the best ways to stimulate the neuroendocrine system and boost these beneficial neurotransmitters, though exercise is a double edged sword. While exercise stimulates these neurotransmitters, it also depletes them, which is a large reason why you feel mental fatigue during exercise. From a dietary standpoint it is obviously imperative to supply your body with adequate carbohydrates to promote an optimal psychological state, but there are also supplements that can potentially improve that state. Most importantly, these supplements can, not only, get you in the zone, but can keep you there longer by minimizing the depletion of these vital neurotransmitters and also by stimulating their release.

TYROSINE

One of these supplements is **tyrosine.** In fact the neurotransmitters epinephrine, norepinephrine and dopamine are all derivatives of the amino acid tyrosine, underscoring the importance of tyrosine for optimal neurological function. Tyrosine at the proper dose has been shown in human studies to improve performance under stressful physiological conditions such as exercise. It can also improve cognitive function, enhancing focus and concentration. Many of these positive attributes of tyrosine are believed to come from its ability to manufacture these neurotransmitters and prevent their depletion during exercise. This makes tyrosine an ideal pre-exercise compound, but only in the proper dosage (2-3 grams) and timing (prior to exercise).

So, now in tyrosine we have and amino acid that supplies the raw material for your body to make performance enhancing neurotransmitters, and we know that exercise itself can release them. But the idea of pre-exercise supplementation for workout enhancement becomes even more interesting when further synergistic compounds are added. One of these compounds, and a very powerful one at that, is **caffeine.**

CAFFEINE

Caffeine stimulates the central nervous system by triggering the release of epinephrine from the adrenal glands and by indirectly blocking a chemical in the body called adenosine, which has calming effects on the central nervous system. Remember, there is an optimal level of central nervous system stimulation, so taking too much of a stimulant can actually worsen performance. Finding the correct dose and ingesting it with proper timing can aid greatly in helping you achieve the optimal state for the most intense and focused training sessions. What's the most effective dose and timing? Research on caffeine shows effective doses in the range of 1.8mg to 4mg per pound of bodyweight, taken about 30 minutes prior to exercise.

BCAA'S

The branch chain amino acids (BCAAs) are crucial for weight trainers looking to increase both anabolism (muscle building) and decrease catabolism (muscle breakdown). But there benefits don't stop there, as research suggests they may also be able to boost performance by fighting central nervous fatigue. While BCAA's potential ability to fight central nervous fatigue is not well understood, one theory referred to as the "central fatigue hypothesis" has emerged as one of the more popular theories.

In a nutshell, the theory looks like this: exercise has shown to increase the tryptophan BCAA ratio, partly due to BCAA's being used as fuel in the muscles during prolonged exercise, depleting their levels. TRP is a precursor to the neurotransmitter serotonin. By exercise depleting BCAA's , there is a possible increase in the tryptophan / BCAA ratio, allowing more tryptophan into the brain, increasing serotonin production. Increased serotonin levels are thought to cause the perception of fatigue to increase and performance to decline.

The theory states that if you increase your BCAA intake, the ratio of tryptophan to BCAA's is decreased and we will experience less fatigue and perform better as a result. Some studies support this theory and show performance gains from BCAA's, while others show no performance gains. Based on the current research, it's difficult to draw firm conclusions if BCAA's do indeed decrease fatigue based on the central fatigue hypothesis. Regardless, you can't go wrong taking BCAA's pre-exercise, as they are beneficial from a muscle building standpoint.

TMG

A final, and very compelling compound is a supplement known as **trimethylglycine (TMG)**, which contains a methyl component that is used to synthesize a substance called SAMe. SAMe, like tyrosine, is also used to make catecholamines such as adrenaline and dopamine. Add it in with tyrosine, caffeine and BCAA's and you have a recipe for increasing mental and physical stimulation, delaying fatigue and increasing exercise performance.

What's Important In a Post-Workout Supplement?

You've nailed it in the gym. You managed to pump out extra reps, pile an extra plate onto your squat and achieve a massive pump in your front quads. As you stagger out the door, you mutter to yourself, "Best work-out ever!"

Your body is now primed to grow. What you put into it in the next hour is going to determine whether that mind blowing workout is going to translate into dense slabs of beef on your frame or whether all of your effort is going to end up being one big waste of time. This, you see, is the critical time for muscle recovery and growth. It's your body's optimum muscle building window. You have to get it right!

The right post workout supplement will allow you to feed your nutrient famished body with just the right combination of carbs and protein in that critical hour after the workout. A post workout supplement may be in the form of tablets, liquid or a shake. It will contain a blend of proteins, carbs, amino acids, vitamins and other ingredients specifically designed to fast track it directly to the muscles that have been stressed during your workout - and provide them with the vital nutrients need to rebuild and repair them, making them bigger and stronger.

Benefits of Using a Post-Workout Supplement

Feed Protein to Depleted Muscle: Confidently fuel your worked muscle with the vital protein it needs, when it needs it.

Recover Quickly: Feed your body with the essential carbs, vitamins and minerals that will allow you to rebound from the workout and get on with your day.

Convenient & Cost-Effective: No hassles preparing food or spending money on high quality lean protein. A supplement is easy and, comparatively, cheap.

Improves Body's Response to Exercise: Allows muscle energy storage to fuel your next workout.

Creatine: Strengthens and rebuilds muscle cells that have been traumatized during the workout

Glutamine: Provides a boost to your body's natural recovery ability.

Post-Workout Must Haves

Whey Protein: Whey is the fastest digesting protein you can consume, which means it delivers its amino acids to your muscles in a hurry to kick-start recovery and muscle growth while the muscles are primed. Speaking of its aminos, it's the richest protein source of the critical BCAA's. Whey also spikes insulin levels, which further promotes muscle growth and helps drive glucose and amino acids into the muscle fibers to aid recovery and growth. Plus, whey has been shown to increase nitric oxide (NO) levels, which can increase blood flow to the recovering muscles to better deliver the nutrients they need after training. Your best bet is a whey protein that offers hydrolyzed whey protein, or whey peptides, along with whey isolate and / or concentrate.

Casein Protein: As good as whey is for quickness, research now confirms that if you back up post-workout whey protein with a very slow digesting protein, muscle growth will be even more impressive than with only whey protein alone. This is likely due to the fact casein provides a slow and steady supply of aminos to the muscles, which keeps muscle protein synthesis turned on for longer and decreases muscle protein breakdown. Your best bet is to use a casein protein that uses a micellar casein; it doesn't mix as well as caseinate, but it's the natural form of casein and digests the slowest. Another good option is a milk protein, such as milk protein isolate or concentrate. Milk protein is 80% casein (the rest is whey), which is maintained in its natural form.

Creatine: This is, without a doubt, the most effective supplement you can use for boosting muscle size and strength. One of the best times to take creatine is right after the workout when your muscle fibers are primed to take up nutrients. Plus, creatine requires insulin for optimal uptake by the muscle fibers. Since, whey protein boosts insulin levels, as do fast digesting carbs, consuming them post-workout with creatine will ensure maximum uptake.

Post-Workout Powerhouses

In addition to the three must-have supplements just discussed, there are a few others you should also consider taking after your workout to truly maximize recovery, growth and strength gains. These four will bump up the results you get with the "must haves" even further.

Carbohydrates: One of the major fuels you burn during your workouts is glycogen, the form of carbohydrates found in your muscle fiber and liver. Doing set after set in the gym depletes muscle glycogen levels, and when they're low muscle recovery and growth are impaired. That's why right after your workout you need a dose of fast digesting carbs, such as dextrose, glucose, maltodextrin and certain high-molecular-weight waxy maize supplements that will get to your muscles within a matter of minutes and restock your muscle glycogen levels so that muscle recovery and growth can continue uncompromised.

These fast digesting carbs also help to spike insulin levels.

Restocking muscle glycogen levels also aids muscle growth in another way. Glycogen pulls water into the muscle cells, causing them to swell, which keeps muscles fuller and larger. This greater fluid volume inside muscle cells places a stretch on muscle fibers that turns on muscle protein synthesis and leads to long term muscle growth. So, make sure to digest some fast digesting carbs after every intense workout.

Beta-Alanine: After your workout, when insulin levels are high, beta alanine rushes into the muscle fiber where it combines with the amino acid histidine to form carnosine. Carnosine helps buffer the acidity level inside muscle fibers so they can contract with more strength for longer periods. Research shows that supplementing with beta-alanine increases muscle strength, power and endurance. And taking it along with creatine has been shown to further boost muscle growth beyond that provided by creatine on its own.

Branch-Chain Amino Acids (BCAA's): These three amino acids - leucine, isoleucine and valine - are the most crucial aminos for muscle growth. Not just because they're used as building blocks to form muscle protein, but because they perform different functions that aid muscle growth. Of the three, leucine is the star; research has discovered that it acts much like the key in the ignition to turn on muscle protein synthesis. This is one reason why the body needs a dose of BCAA's immediately after workouts. Another reason is because all three have been shown to work together to blunt cortisol levels after training. When you finish training, your body gets flooded with a cascade of hormones. Some of these hormones, such as testosterone, are anabolic. Others, like cortisol, are catabolic. Cortisol also interferes with testosterone, lowering its levels and its ability to drive muscle growth. The goal after workouts is to maximize testosterone levels and minimize cortisol. This is precisely what BCAA's do when added to a post-workout shake.

If you take a 40 gram dose of protein from a combination of whey and casein, it should deliver close to four grams of leucine. However, if you truly want to ensure that muscle protein synthesis is maxed, you'll want to add some extra BCAA's post-workout.

Glutamine: This amino acid is another one that can really help after workouts. Glutamine aids in the recovery of muscle glycogen. It can help more of the carbs you're consuming get stored as glycogen in muscle fibers. Glutamine also boosts growth hormone (GH) levels, which is important after workouts to encourage greater muscle growth and strength gains. Another reason it's important to take glutamine after training is to maintain immune function. Tough workouts can deplete muscle glutamine levels and compromise your immune system, making you more susceptible to colds and other minor illnesses. A dose of glutamine will keep your immune system in tip-top condition, helping to prevent you from getting sick and missing workouts.

Creating the Ultimate Anabolic Environment

Putting yourself in a positive anabolic environment will allow your body to fuel your muscle cells for maximum size and strength. Adding stress in the form of weight training will allow you to start building that muscle. However, there is a hormone that your body naturally releases as a result of stress that can stop you building muscle. And, it's released when you put yourself under the stress of weight training.

It's called cortisol.

However, there is a solution. It's called Phosphatidylesrine or PS. PS can block the release of cortisol and prevent its catabolic (muscle devouring) effects. In theory this supplement has the potential to positively affect important hormones that can help you put on muscle. But it doesn't work the same way a pro-hormone or testosterone booster works. PS works in a completely different manner.

Cortisol is a glucocorticoid and is catabolic. This means it takes proteins, amino acids and fatty acids and breaks them down into smaller molecules in order to produce glucose, which is the body's preferred energy source and the only source for certain vital functions - for example the brain cannot use anything but glucose for energy. Cortisol gets a bad rap because it takes the proteins and amino acids that the body needs directly from your muscles.

That's only half the story though - cortisol does other things. If you lose the ability to produce cortisol, you don't magically gain muscle. In fact, people that don't produce any cortisol have little muscle and very weak bodies because cortisol is crucial for maintaining a healthy immune system (if the immune system isn't working right, the last thing that the body is worried about is maintaining "showy" muscles that aren't necessary for survival). The point here is that the body needs some cortisol.

The concern with high levels of cortisol is that muscle mass is very difficult to build when it's constantly being broken down and converted into glucose. Resistance exercise is one activity that can have a protective effect on your muscles by preventing cortisol from working as effectively (lifting weights weakens cortisol's ability to bind to proteins in your muscle cells). The hormonal environment of your muscle cells plays a large role in determining whether or not a muscle cell grows or atrophies (shrinks) and so by tipping the scales in favor of a more anabolic environment (by reducing cortisol levels and increasing testosterone levels) it becomes much more likely that you will be able to put on muscle. Even though weight training may prevent cortisol from doing some of its work, if cortisol levels are chronically elevated, then muscular gains will be compromised. An ideal situation would be to raise testosterone (an anabolic hormone) and lower cortisol (a catabolic hormone). This is where PS comes in because it can do both.

PS Evidence

In one study, 11 weight trained men were exposed to a placebo-treatment condition and a PS treatment condition. During the placebo condition they received something that should not have induced any changes in hormone levels, while during the treatment condition they received 800 mg of PS per day. The subjects performed 5 sets of 10 reps of 13 exercises, 4 times a week for 2 weeks. This protocol was followed for both treatment conditions. After 6 days of PS supplementation, cortisol levels decreased and testosterone levels increased. These results were in agreement with earlier studies which showed PS could decrease cortisol levels. There was almost a 50% reduction in cortisol levels and 30% increase in testosterone during the times described above. This could be interpreted as a very favorable environment for muscle growth - primarily due to the dramatic decrease in cortisol levels. This phenomenon has been observed in heavy steroid users because steroids occupy the same cell sites as cortisol, thus preventing catabolism (muscle breakdown). (3)

Another benefit regarding PS supplementation includes improved wellbeing and lower levels of muscle soreness (less duration and intensity). This can be very good for muscle growth because it will allow you to recover faster from hard training sessions - you won't have soreness that may hold you back from training other body parts with maximum intensity.

Other effects of PS include improved ability to concentrate, improvements in short term memory and improved scores in neuropsychological tests. Most of these studies were initially done on elderly people but recent evidence shows that the results are applicable to younger people as well. For example, tests examining brain activity in younger adults found substantial increases in EEG (electro-encephalogram) reading after PS supplementation indicating increased brain activity caused by improved neural functioning.

A concern regarding PS supplementation is that the long term uses of PS have not been studied. Lower cortisol levels may be beneficial to a point, but what if this develops into an inability to respond to stress? There is no real evidence one way or another. However, after swallowing a couple of capsules of PS, it crosses the gastrointestinal tract, enters your bloodstream and gets incorporated into your cells. The PS is placed on an inner portion of the cell membrane and helps to maintain membrane fluidity. This portion of the cell is very dynamic and is subject to change based upon a person's diet, but there is no evidence of long term negative effects with PS via this mechanism. Once you go off it, the body should revert back to its previous normal state.

Lowering Cortisol Naturally

There are other things you can do to lower your cortisol levels and, therefore, help to create the ultimate anabolic environment. Cortisol is sensitive to many things. Lack of sleep, excess protein and stress of any kind all affect cortisol levels in one way or another. To lower cortisol levels naturally, get plenty of sleep, don't get too worked up over things, spend time doing things that relax you, keep dietary carbohydrates higher than protein intake for all meals and, most importantly, avoid overtraining. Keeping a training journal and tracking your progress is a good way to prevent overtraining. If things are not improving you may be doing something wrong - possibly overdoing it.

PS can help improve your training. It will allow you to handle higher workloads without overtaxing your recovery abilities. By handling higher workloads, you get a better training effect. This means more muscle size and strength down the road, assuming diet and recovery time are sufficient.

PS Dosage

The dosage to take appears to be 800mg per day as used in previous studies (400 mg in the morning and 400mg at night). Taking more may be beneficial for muscle growth, but could cause other problems - if your cortisol levels get too low, then your joints may start to ache (in this case more probably isn't better). If your cortisol levels are lowered, just shy of experiencing any joint pain and you are taking a pro hormone, you should get a nice increase in the testosterone to cortisol ratio and avoid any problems.(4)

Chapter 11: Customizing Your Supplements

There are thousands of supplements on the market, each offering stellar results. The following essentials guide will allow you to cut through the advertising hoop-la and zero in on the exact supplements that you need for your specific goals.

Strength And Power Boosters

Beta-alanine

Beta-alanine is an amino acid that is naturally produced in the body. It is not, therefore, an essential amino acid. Its muscle building benefit lies in its ability to aid in the synthesis of carnosine, which is a dipeptide found within muscle fiber. As a result, it has been shown to reduce muscle fatigue and enhance overall workout capacity as well as boosting explosive muscle strength. With beta-alanine you'll be able to train harder for longer.

Recommendation: Consume 5g of beta-alanine daily just prior to your workout.

Creatine

Creatine is a naturally occurring nutrient found in meat and fish. It can be produced in the body by the liver and pancreas from the amino acids arginine, glycine and methionine. 95% of creatine is stored within muscle cells. During high intensity training your body relies on phosphocreatine to resynthesize ATP. Once these stores are exhausted, performance begins to decline. Creatine supplementation increases stores of phosphocreatine, allowing your muscles to work at higher rates for a longer time. This will produce an immediate strength boost.

Recommendation: Use a loading protocol, involving consuming .3 g per kg of body weight for 3-5 days, followed by 3-5g after that. Take in combination with protein and carbs. Take immediately prior to your work-out.

Betaine

Betaine is a derivative of the non-essential amino acid glycine. It is synthesized naturally within the body. Dietary sources of Betaine include wheat, beets, spinach and shellfish. Recent studies suggest that it may help to facilitate hydration, increase strength, enhance endurance and improve work-out recovery. There is also some suggestion that supplementation with Betaine enhances fat metabolism.

Recommendation: Take 4g of betaine prior to your work-out. Betaine comes in either powder, tablet or capsule form.

Energy Boosters

Tyrosine

Tyrosine is a non-essential amino acid, meaning that it can be produced within the body. It is easily obtainable from high-protein foods such as soy, turkey, chicken, fish, peanuts, almonds and dairy foods. It is used in the production of protein and is a key precursor of the neurotransmitter dopamine. Dopamine acts in concert with serotonin. When they are out of balance, fatigue ensues. Supplementation with Tyrosine helps to maintain the body's balance between dopamine and serotonin. The result is reduced fatigue and enhanced performance.

Recommendation: Take 150 mg per kg of body-weight one hour before your work-out. A 100kg would, therefore, take 9.5 g per day.

Taurine

Taurine is a sulfur-containing non-essential amino acid. One of the most abundant amino acids in the body, it is found in muscle and organ tissue. Taurine is found naturally in fish, beef, poultry and lamb. It is a popular ingredient in energy drinks such as Red Bull. Taurine is believed to affect cellular excitability by increasing the release of calcium from the sarcoplasmic reticulum. This allows for greater actin and myosin interaction, thus improving muscle contractibility and force production. Taurine also combats oxidative free radicals that are produced during exercise. Supplementing with Taurine before and during your workout, will delay fatigue and improve performance by improving strength and power during muscle contraction.

Recommendation: Take 1-2 g of Taurine per day prior to your work-out. It would probably pay to avoid the Red Bull, however. Although each can contains 1 g of Taurine, it comes with a whole heap of sugar.

Rhodiola Rosea

Rhodiola Rosea is a herbal plant that grows in the mountainous regions of central and northern Europe, Asia and North America as well as in the cold climate of the Arctic. Rhodiola Rosea is thought to have a beneficial effect on energy usage. It does this by increasing essential energy metabolites, ATP, and creatine phosphate within muscle and brain mitochondria. This process also boosts fat metabolism.

Recommendation: Take 250 mg of Rhodiola Rosea twice daily, in the morning and early afternoon.

Ginseng

Ginseng refers to extracts derived from the plant family Araliacae. Ginseng has been touted for a broad range of aliments from AIDS to zoster. In traditional Chinese medicine it is used to restore Qi, or life energy. It is often consumed as a tonic for vitality, health, longevity, strength, wisdom and general wellbeing. Athletes take ginseng to improve physical and athletic stamina or as a herbal support during rigorous training.

Most side effects of ginseng use are mild and reversible when they do occur. Causal relationships often cannot be established in combination products that contain ginseng as one of the main ingredients.

Recommendation: Generally dosage is around 0.6 to 3 grams of root powder 1 to 3 times per day for Panax ginseng, and as a capsule or extract standardized to 4-8% ginsenosides, 200-400 mg per day. Sometimes ginseng is taken continuously, but cycling is usually recommended.

Schisandra Chinensis

Schisandra Chinensis is a herb derived from a vine that is native to Russia and China. It has been used for centuries as a Chinese medical cure-all. The Western world has recently come to appreciate the benefits of this herb in terms of its ability to support muscle endurance and to control cortisol levels.

Recommendation: As there are not yet any Western clinical studies on Schisandra Chinensis it is not possible to provide dosage guidelines.

B Vitamins

The B Vitamins consist of the following 8 water soluble vitamins: Thiamine, Riboflavin,

Niacin, Pyridoxine, Folic acid, Pantothenic acid, Biotin, B 12. All 8 vitamins work together to provide a host of health benefits, including increasing the rate of metabolism, maintaining high energy levels and enhancing fat digestion.

Recommendation: Take a complex B vitamin that contains at least 10 mg of B12 in the morning.

Stimulants

Caffeine

Caffeine is a chemical compound found in over 60 species of plants, including coffee beans, tea leaves, cocoa beans, guarana and kola nuts. 45 - 60 minutes after ingestion, a number of physiological responses occur that allow a person to remain alert with a clearer flow of thought, increased focus and better general body coordination. Caffeine also increases fat oxidation. This helps to spare muscle glycogen and wards off premature muscle fatigue.

Recommendations: Take 5-7 mg of caffeine per kg of bodyweight.

Yerba Mate

Yerba Mate is an ancient beverage that is made from the leaves of the small evergreen holly tree, which is found in several South American countries. Yerbe Mate is well known throughout South America for its health giving properties. Blending caffeine and antioxidants, Yerbe provides a natural energy boost that can help power you through your workouts. In addition this wonder compound provides 24 vitamins and minerals and 15 different amino acids. In all, it contains 196 health giving compounds.

Recommendation: Take a cup of Yerbe Mate 30 minutes prior to your workout.

Muscle Builders

Branched-Chain Amino Acids

Branch-Chain Amino Acids (BCAAs), include the amino acids leucine, isoleucine and valine. All three of these are considered essential amino acids because they are not synthesized by the body and must, therefore be supplied by our diet. BCAA's are unique in that they can be oxidized in the muscles for fuel. The other essential amino acids are broken down in the liver. BCAA's, especially leucine, are key stimulators of protein synthesis and protein breakdown. BCAA's can be used as fuel during exercise. They will also prevent the catabolic effects of working out. Post-workout they can enhance muscle building effects.

Recommendations: Most experts recommend a slightly higher dosage of leucine and smaller dosages of valine and isoleucine. Supplement with 8g of BCAAs daily in a ratio of leucine / valine isoleucine of 3:1:1

Glutamine

Glutamine is the most abundant amino acid found in the human body. It is mainly synthesized and stored in muscles. Heavy weight training is associated with drops in blood glutamine levels, increasing susceptibility to infection . As well as providing athletes with immune support, glutamine supplementation promotes protein synthesis and help prevent muscle breakdown. Glutamine can be especially helpful to trainers who are experiencing burn-out or overtraining.

Recommendation: Glutamine is available in tablet, capsule and powder form. It should be taken pre (30 minutes prior to the workout), during and post workout at a dosage of 4g.

Carnitine

Although often referred to as an amino acid, Carnitine is actually an amino-like compound that is formed in the body by the amino acids lysine and methionine. Carnitine (which comes from the Latin word for meat) is abundant in red meat, dairy foods, nuts, grains and green vegetables. Carnitine assists the body to transport fat into the mitochondria of cells. It is in the mitochondria that the fat is burned as fuel. In addition, Carnitine assists in blood flow by increasing nitric oxide (NO) production.

Recommendation: To achieve the muscle enhancing effects that you need, Carnitine requires insulin. For this reason, supplementation should be done in conjunction with a high carb meal or with your protein shake. A daily dosage of 2-33 g is ideal.

Pump Providers

Citrulline Malate

Citrulline malate is a the result of the bonding of the non-essential amino-acid citrulline with the organic salt compound malate. By itself citrulline is synthesized from the amino acid glutamine within the intestines. It plays an important part in the removal of ammonia, which is a by-product of exercise that can negatively affect the production of energy, leading to fatigue and reduced performance. Malate is found naturally in fruits such as apples and plays a role in the series of chemical reactions known as the Krebs cycle, which produces energy from carbohydrates, fats and protein. Malate is also able to recycle lactate for energy production. This is critical in maintaining the muscles from fatigue and aiding recovery. Acting together, Citrulline and malate enhance training performance by accelerating the clearance of fatigue-inducing ammonia and recycling lactate for improved energy production.

Recommendation: Take 2-3g 30 minutes before your workout and another 2-3 grams at bedtime, preferably on an empty stomach.

Arginine

Arginine is what is known as a conditionally essential amino acid. Our bodies are capable of synthesizing arginine, but under certain conditions (trauma, disease, stress) the body cannot produce enough, making dietary sources essential. Arginine can be found in foods such as nuts, seeds, beans, fish and chicken. Arginine can be metabolized into glucose for energy during exercise. It is also important in the production of nitric oxide and creatine. In addition, arginine has been shown to stimulate the production of growth hormone, a powerful muscle building stimulant.

Recommendation: Take 7-9 g of arginine daily.

GPLC

Glycine Propionyl-L-Carnitine (GPLC) consists of a molecular bonded form of propionyl-L-carnitine and the carnitine precursor amino acid glycine. Recent studies have shown that supplementation with GPLC enhances blood flow while working out. This was achieved by increasing levels of nitric oxide (NO). All of this will allow for a greater pump during workouts as nutrients are more readily transported to the working muscle. GPLC has also been reported to reduce workout fatigue and enhance endurance due to the increased ability of nutrients to get to the working muscle.

Recommendation: Take 4.5 g of GLPC 30 minutes before your workout.

Pycnogenol

Pycnogenol is a herbal extract derived from the bark of a French maritime pine tree. It contains plant compounds called oligomeric proanthocyanidin complexes (OPCs), which carry strong antioxidant qualities that improve recovery times during heavy training sessions. Pycnogenol is also believed to help inhibit the enzymes responsible for the destruction of lung tissue in bronchitis sufferers. It does this by decreasing the amount of circulating inflammatory substances in the blood stream. This substance also reduces muscle pain as a result of heavy training.

Recommendation: Take 2.4 g of Pycnogenol with water 4 hours before your workout. Pycnogenol is available in tablet and capsule form.

Nitrates

Nitrates are a naturally occurring form of nitrogen found in soil. As a result they are found in foods produced from the ground. An abundant source of nitrates is the beetroot. Nitrates have been shown to boost nitric oxide (NO) production which results in greater exercise endurance, greater power potential and less fatigue.

Recommendation: Take 500 mg of beet extract 30 minutes prior to your workout.

Glycerol

Glycerol is a sugar alcohol that is colorless, odorless and sweet tasting. Glycerol is sourced from oils and fats and is used to retain moisture from the air. Because of its water retention properties, glycerine has a hydrating effect on the body. It can, therefore, help a bodybuilder to dry out and achieve that shrink wrapped look prior to going on stage. It can also counter the negative effects of dehydration while training. Interestingly, glycerol is often added to health bars as a sweetener. Because it is officially classed as a carbohydrate, it boosts up the carb count of the bar without adding the energy boost that one might expect when reading the label.

Recommendation: Take 1 g per kg of bodyweight an hour before working out.

Brain Boosters

Choline

Choline is a member of the B-vitamin family. High fat meats such as beef liver, as well as chicken, milk, soybeans and eggs are excellent sources of choline. It has a number of significant roles in the body, including neurotransmitter synthesis, cell membrane signaling, lipid transport and homocysteine metabolism. Significantly for weight trainers, choline acts as a precursor in acetylcholine synthesis with a vital role in muscle contraction. It binds to receptors on muscles and it is this binding which activates muscle contraction.

Recommendation: Take 2.5 g of choline one hour prior to your workout.

Dimethylmylamine (DMAE)

Dimethylmylamine (DMAE) is a pharmaceutical amphetamine derivative. It can be found in over 200 sports supplements. DMAE has strong stimulatory effects on the body. Scientists don't know exactly how it works, but many speculate that it binds to sympathetic nervous system or adrenal receptors, initiating a strong sympathetic response increasing heart rate, heightening alertness and increasing the force produced within the muscles. It also appears that DMAE increases metabolic rate with a resultant enhanced fat burning effect.

Huperzine A

Huperzine A is a derivative of the Chinese club moss plant. On its journey to supplement form, Huperzine A goes through quite a bit of laboratory manipulation. It has been proven to be beneficial for memory and learning enhancement, and is especially beneficial for helping to reverse the effects of Alzheimer's Disease. Huperzine A is also beneficial in boosting the immune system.

Recommendation: Huperzine A is available in liquid, tablet and capsule form. Take 50 mg with breakfast.

Fat Burners

Green Tea Extract

Green Tea Extract is an extract of green tea leaves. It contains antioxidants mainly in the form of green tea polyphenols and catechins as well as caffeine, all of which are believed to aid fat loss by inducing thermogenesis, stimulating fat oxidation and increasing metabolism.

Recommendation: Green Tea extract is available as a drink and in capsule form. Simply taking it in the form of a cup of green tea makes most sense, as it will not only allow you to take in about 50 mg of caffeine and 100 mg of polyphenol, it also offers hydration in the form of water. And, if you daily replace your mocachino with green tea, you'll be sparing hundreds of calories in the process.

Synephrine

Synephrine is a proto-alkaloid found in bitter orange extract, which is derived from citrus fruits such as seville, mandarins, sweet oranges, tangerines and grapefruits. Structurally, synephrine is similar to ephedrine, which was banned by the United

States Food and Drug Administration (FDA) in 2003 as a result of negative health concerns.

A variety of cells within the body have alpha and beta adrenal receptors. These adrenal receptors are targets for stress hormones and catecholamines released in response to exercise, such as epinephrine and norepinephrine, which initiate the fight or flight response. This binding induces a strong sympathetic response including increased heart rate, heightened alertness and increased force production within the muscles - all of which allow the body to overcome stress. This response increases metabolic rate and subsequent fat oxidation. Alkaloids such as synephrine and ephedrine, like catecholamine, can bind these receptors and induce a sympathetic response, potentially increasing resting metabolic rate and fat oxidation. As a result synephrine is often added to weight loss supplements.

Recommendation: Take 45 g per day.

Yohimbe

Yohimbe is an evergreen tree native to Zaire, Cameroon and Gabon. The bark of the tree contains the chemical yohimbine. Yohimbine was believed for some time to enhance testosterone levels, but this has been proven to be false. It has, however, proven itself as a libido enhancer and cure-all for erectile dysfunction. Although not scientifically proven, it appears that yohimbine may also be beneficial in helping to remove the stubborn fat that typically stores itself around the waist of men and the hips and thighs of women.

Recommendation: Yohimbe carries it with the side effect of anxiety in higher dosages. It is important, to then, keep the dosage manageable. Take .2 mg per kg of bodyweight.

Spotlight on Human Growth Hormone

Human growth hormone can turn back your body's internal clock, helping you rapidly build muscle, slash fat and increase libido, all while sending energy levels through the roof. Still there's lot of confusion surrounding this powerful anabolic hormone. Here are answers to some common questions.

Question: What is human growth hormone?

Answer: The body naturally produces growth hormone in the pituitary gland and, as its name implies, it is responsible for cell growth and regeneration. Increasing muscle mass and bone density are impossible without human growth hormone. However, it is also a major player in maintaining the health of all human tissue, including that of the brain and other vital organs. The secreted growth hormone remains active in the bloodstream for only a few minutes, but this is enough time for the liver to convert it into growth factors, the most critical of which is insulin-like growth factor-1 or IGF-1. IGF-1 boosts a host of anabolic properties. Scientists began to harvest growth hormone from the pituitary glands of cadavers in the 1950's, but didn't synthesize the first human growth hormone in laboratories until 1981, with its use as a performance enhancing drug becoming popular thereafter.

Question: How much growth hormone do I produce naturally?

Answer: Healthy adult men typically have just less than 5 nanograms per milliliter circulating in the blood. Healthy females can produce about twice that amount for child bearing purposes. Levels for both sexes peak during puberty and drop sharply during the early 20's.

Question: How can I learn if I have a GH deficiency?

Answer: Ask your doctor to perform a growth hormone test. You'll need to fast for a simple blood test.

Question: Age related declines are natural. Why do I need growth hormone if I'm not growing anymore?

Answer: Aside from growth hormone's crucial role in building muscle mass, not all of its benefits are necessarily evident to the naked eye. Growth hormone has been shown to slow the progression of age-related degenerative diseases as well as increase sex drive, help mental acuity, and engender a general sense of wellbeing. The flip side of the coin - low growth hormone - can result in the exact opposite; muscle loss, fat gain, low sex drive and energy levels, and a poor sense of wellbeing.

Question: How can I boost growth hormone levels?

Answer: Two major factors that contribute to increased growth hormones levels are ones you can control without drugs - weight training exercise and sleep. The more you exercise the more growth hormone you release naturally. A recent study observed significant increases in circulating growth hormone and IGF-1 after intense resistance exercise in a group of trained men but found no significant differences in untrained men who performed the same workout. Growth hormone is also secreted while you sleep, and studies have shown a spike in growth hormone levels at the onset of deep sleep, so getting the recommended seven to nine hours per night is essential to maintain growth hormone. Diet is the third major factor in keeping growth hormone levels topped off. It is necessary to eat a balanced diet that provides as many of the following growth hormone boosting agents as possible:

Vitamin A

Vitamin B5

Vitamin B12

Folic Acid

Inositol Heaxanicotinate

Chromium

Zinc

Magnesium

Iodine

Glutamine

Glycine

Carnitine

Arginine

Taurine

Lysine

Ornithine Alpha-ketoglutarate

Question: What supplements can I take to boost growth hormone?

Answer: A multivitamin provides many of the nutrients needed to boost growth hormone. Amino acids such as arginine and glutamine have been shown to boost growth hormone levels in separate studies. Instead of taking these separately, you now have the choice between a multitude of specialty supplements.

Other hormones, such as testosterone, estrogen, progesterone, can also lead to growth hormone increases. The following compounds have all been shown to enhance growth hormone levels;

Colostrum

Alpha GPC

Tribulus terrestris

Coleus forskohlii

Panax ginseng

Siberian ginseng

Aswagandha root

Schizandra berry

Astragalus root

Dong quai

Wild yam extract

Goji berry

Red date berry

Creating the Ultimate Stack

Back in the day, bodybuilding nutrition consisted of little more than some protein powder and a blender. Today, however, it's much more complex. The "craze" for size and the fastest possible gains has led supplement scientists deeper into the labs seeking more and more scientifically backed compounds and formulations.

The outcome of such research has given us countless high-tech additives and new super supplements, all of which promise to push your gains from average to explosive. As exciting as today's store shelves appear, unfortunately the expansion of products has made choosing which ones to use that much more difficult.

You've no doubt walked into your local health and supplement store and within seconds realized that devising any supplement regime can be a daunting task, never mind one that best suits your own personal needs. By simply grabbing whatever the sales guy recommends off the shelf, you risk taking the entire "kitchen sink" home, instead of just the products that you need. The following stack are scientifically compiled to meet a complete spectrum of bodybuilding goals, from getting lean to building maximum muscle, repairing joint health to boosting testosterone and growth hormone levels, improving sleep and softening the effects of estrogen.

Lean Mass Stack

The Stack : Whey Protein Isolate; Creatine Monohydrate; Honey

A good quality whey protein isolate (WPI) is crucial in your supplement regime when you're trying to add lean mass. Not only does it provide a complete array of amino acids to promote anabolism, it helps boost your immune system and aids in fat loss. Creatine monohydrate (CM) on the other hand, acts as a cell volumizer by increasing water and increasing glycogen resynthesis, which helps to replenish muscular levels of creatine for short term energy. It also increases insulin-like growth factor-1 (IGF-1) and has a myriad of other health benefits supported by over two decades of scientific data.

Honey is a fairly even mix of glucose and fructose, the latter of which actually makes it a relatively slow digesting carb, perfect for fueling a workout. It's commonly known that glucose (simple and fast digesting) triggers a significant elevation in blood insulin levels, which acts as a potent anabolic stimulant. Many are on the fence, however, when it comes to adding sugars to their diet (mainly due to fear of gaining unwanted weight). Yet, a recent study out of Australia has shown that consuming whey protein, creatine and carbohydrates together leads to significant increases in strength and lean mass (compared to whey alone or a combination of whey and carbs). (5)

Dosage:

Drink three of these shakes per day. For optimal results, consume one when you wake up, one before working out and the third one before working out, and the third one before going to bed. Each shake should contain 20-40 grams of WPI, 3-5 grams of CM (based on you tolerance levels and 35 grams (approx. 2 tablespoons) of honey. Mix these ingredients in a blender with 470 mls of water.

Pre and Post Training Strength Stack

The Stack: Creatine Monohydrate; Beta-Alanine and Arginine; Alpha-Ketoglutarate (AAKG)

Beta-alanine, which is a non-essential amino acid found in protein rich foods, has been shown to increase muscle carnosine levels by

60% in as little as 2-4 weeks and by greater than 80% after only 10 weeks. Carnosine buffers exercise related metabolic by-products that lead to fatigue. And, as is the case with creatine, arginine alpha-ketoglutarate (AAKG) has also been shown to boost strength. It promotes vasodilation (widening of blood vessels) during exercise and subsequently augments nutrient delivery and metabolic clearance. Additionally AAKG has been shown to increase plasma levels of several strength associated hormones such as growth hormone (GH), insulin, norepineephrine and epinephrine.

Dosage:

Mix 3-5 grams of CM, 2 grams of beta-alanine and 2-5 grams of AAKG into a 275 ml drink containing glucose (fast acting sugars) such as Kool-Aid or Gatorade. Drink one serving 30 minutes before training and another serving immediately after your workout.

Growth Hormone (GH) Releasing Stack

The Stack: Mucuna Pruriens; L-Arginine: Fenugreek

Mucuna pruriens has been shown to significantly increase L-dopa, which is required to augment GH release. L-arginine and fenugreek seeds are also scientifically backed as GH secretagogues (releasing agents). GH is a potent stimulator of both muscular growth and fat loss, and thus has a significant positive impact on body composition. Together these supplements potentiate (or enhance) natural GH release through several different pathways in your body. (6)

Dosage:

Combine 2 grams of mucuna pruriens extract (look for products that are standardized for a minimum of 15% L-dopa), 2-5 grams of L-arginine (based on tolerance level) and 0.5-1 gram of fenugreek seed extract; mix with 275 mls of water. Consume immediately before going to bed and again upon waking.

Sleep Stack

The Stack: Micellar Casein Protein; ZMA; Gamma-Aminobutyric Acid: 5-Hydroxytryptophan

Compared to all available proteins, micellar casein is the superior bedtime option. It provides a steady release of amino acids into the bloodstream for up to seven hours, and thus best defends against catabolism (muscle breakdown) while you sleep. Combined with ZMA (a form of zinc), which has been shown to increase IGF-1 and testosterone levels, these supplements promote an anabolic sleep environment. The inhibitory CNS neurotransmitter gamma-aminobutyric acid (GABA) and 5-Hydorxytryptophan (5-HTP), which is a precursor to serotonin, both promote healthy and deep sleep required for GH release, muscular recovery and growth.

Dosage:

Several foods can alter the absorption of zinc based products; as such, ZMA should be taken (as per label directions on the bottle) at least one hour after consuming your last meal and one hour prior to ingesting the remainder of this stack. Combine 30-50 grams of micellar casein protein with 1-3 grams of GABA and 50-100 milligrams of 5-HTP. Mix all the ingredients with 475 mls of water. For best results, consume this shake immediately before going to bed.

Cell Volumizing Stack:

The Stack: Creatine; Glutamine; l-Arginine: Waxy Maize

Several studies show that glutamine and creatine mixed with a fast digesting carbohydrate (such as dextrose, maltodextrin or waxy maize) results in dramatic increases in muscular volume (size). Unlike dextrose or maltodextrin, however, waxy maize is not a sugar. Though it's still considered a fast-digesting carb, compared to other sources, it's able to bypass the stomach, be absorbed by the intestines and go to work much quicker. Arginine on the other hand, is a well-known intermediary needed to promote vasodilation (widening of blood vessels).

Taken together, these supplements act to rapidly and potently increase your muscle pump and enhance muscle cell volume. This effect will not only make you to look bigger while working out, but will also provide a powerful stimulus for muscle hypertrophy (growth) over the long term. (7)

Dosage:

Combine 3-5 grams of your favorite form of creatine, 3-5 grams of L-glutamine, 3-5 grams of L-arginine and 30 grams of waxy maize (check label instructions as some products recommend consuming it as a standalone supplement). Mix this with 475 mls of water (you may want to add flavor and crystals to it) or add it to your pre-workout protein shake. Consume one serving 30 minutes before training and another immediately after.

Testosterone Booster Pack

The Stack: Tribulus Terrestris; Tongkat Ali: Fenugreek

Testosterone increases protein synthesis and muscle growth. Together tribulus terrestris, tongkat ali and fenugreek (plant extracts)have been scientifically proven to boost testosterone production and release the hormone via several different mechanisms.

Dosage:

Several supplement manufacturers have already combined these herbal extracts into one formulation. However, be sure to watch for products that list the percentage of standardization of extracts. These products should contain no less than 80% total saponins and at least 40% protodioscin. Take the product as per label directions, and cycle five days on and two days off for a maximum of four weeks. After a two week recovery you may resume cycling in the same manner.

Energizer Stack

The Stack: Yerba Mate; Caffeine Anhydrous; Xanthinol Nicotinate; Citrulline Malate

Yerba mate and caffeine are potent central nervous system (CNS) stimulants that have been scientifically proven to increase alertness, focus and exercise intensity. Xanthinol Nicotinate is a form of niacin (vitamin B3) that increases brain and muscle blood flow and brain glucose metabolism, and it also leads to increased exercise tolerance. Citrulline malate is a potent form of citrulline (a non-essential amino acid) that combats exercise fatigue, increases time to exhaustion and aids in the production of arginine (a precursor to nitric oxide) to promote greater blood flow in muscle tissue. Take this stuff 30 minutes before working out and you should be able to push harder, with more intensity, and for a longer period of time.

Dosage:

Yerba mate is available in many forms, such as tea, powder and capsule, and contains a modest amount of caffeine. Generally one serving of powdered extract is 2-3 grams. Combine this with 3-5 grams of citrulline malate and then mix with 240 mls of water (add sweetener if desired). Caffeine anhydrous is most easily consumed in tablet form; take 200-300 mg (based on your tolerance level) along with the yerbe mate / citrulline malate drink, followed by 150-300 mg of xanthinol nicotinate.

Anti-Estrogen Stack

The Stack: Androstenetrione; Diindolymethane

The accumulation of estrogen, a female hormone, can lead to increases in body fat storage, not to mention water retention. Even worse, however, is that testosterone converts to estrogen when it encounters enzymes known as aromatases. Androstenetrione and diindolymethane (DIM) act as natural aromatase inhibitors, blocking the conversion of testosterone to estrogen, thus promoting lower estrogen levels and higher circulating testosterone levels.

Dose:

Consume 200-400 mg of androstenetrione and 100-400 mg of diindolymethane with your last meal of the day. Cycle this stack six weeks on and four weeks off.

General Health Stack

The Stack: Whey Protein Isolate; Multivitamin / Mineral Supplement; Fish Oil; Chromium Picolinate

High quality whey protein isolate products contain large amounts of immune system boosting enzymes and protein fractions (such as beta lactoglobulin, alpha lactalbumin and immunoglobulin) each of which offers its own benefits. Although most protein products also contain vitamin / mineral additives, a standalone multivitamin / mineral supplement ensures that when your body is physically stressed, it receives all of the macronutrients needed to function optimally, Fish oils contain Omega-3 fatty acids that are scientifically proven to protect the heart and reduce cholesterol, support brain function and healthy body composition, and, as with

WPI, help to boost the immune system. Keeping your insulin levels in check is also important for good health. Chromium picolinate not only stabilizes blood sugar levels, but also aids in fat loss.

Dose:

Immediately upon waking, ingest 20-40 grams of whey protein isolate mixed with 450 mls of water to stave off catabolism and boost immune system function. Along with your shake, ingest the multivitamin / mineral supplement (as per label instructions), 100-2000 mg of high quality fish oil and 200 micrograms of chromium picolinate. Then, consume a solid breakfast within 30 minutes. You should also take 1,000-2,000 mg of fish oil and 300 micrograms of chromium picolinate with both lunch and dinner.

Testosterone Boosters

Testosterone, and it's "chemical cousins" anabolic steroids, are powerful muscle-building and performance enhancing compounds. For well over half a century they have been the secret weapon behind many world class athlete's performances and played a significant role in the history of bodybuilding.

Steroids and testosterone increase the amount of muscle you can build. Steroids, however, have side effects. Some of them are not do serious, other are very serious. Steroids are also banned by virtually every athletic organization and are controlled substances. If you get busted buying or selling them on the black market or smuggling them in from other countries where they are sold over the counter (like Mexico) you can find yourself doing hard time.

As many as three million athletes in the United States alone have used anabolic steroids in the last 10 years. Yet, scientific research and exciting new theories have put us on the cusp of making illegal anabolic steroids all but obsolete.

Testosterone: Natural VS Synthetic

Testosterone that is naturally produced in your body is safer than synthetic testosterone made in a lab. It took hundreds of thousands of years to develop the hormonal cascades that shower our bodies with natural testosterone. Scientist have known how to scientifically manufacture testosterone for about 60 years now, but a mere 6 decades cannot catch up with hundreds of thousands of years of natural development.

If we can naturally boost testosterone levels, we won't need to take synthetic drugs to get the extra edge. Fortunately, new, ground breaking scientific theories offer strong evidence that it is, indeed, possible to naturally, and significantly, elevate your testosterone levels by using a precise combination of novel dietary supplements.

Some of the most powerful testosterone boosters, which have become extremely popular among bodybuilders recently, are androstenedione, tribulus terrestris and DHEA. Even though most serious weight trainers already know about these supplements, many are unsure about the specifics of how to best utilize them.

DHEA

DHEA is a mild androgenic pro-hormone naturally produced in the body by the adrenal glands. It's two steps up the metabolic pathway from testosterone, meaning that one of its metabolic fates is to be converted to testosterone in the body.

Because supplemental forms of DHEA were originally targeted to older adults to help reverse the dwindling DHEA and testosterone levels common to that population, much of the research has been done with subjects over the age of 50. These studies show supplementation with between 50 and 100 mg per day in men and women over 50 may be able to return blood DHEA levels similar to those of young adults, increase immune cell function, and even help build muscle size and strength and burn more body fat.

As word of these studies spread, DHEA use caught on among bodybuilders and other athletes looking for a testosterone boost. Unfortunately, there is very little research available on the effects of DHEA in young, active individuals. One study showed taking a whopping 1,600 mg per day helped subjects lose 31% of their body fat in only 28 days, while concurrently putting on muscle mass. (8)

Although research in athletes is lacking, DHEA may prove useful to serious iron pumpers. Intense training may lead to suppression of testosterone production. Supplying excess hormone substrate (such as DHEA) may help counter some of this effect and support higher testosterone production and blood levels.

Androstenedione: The East German Secret Weapon

If DHEA is the one that started it all, androstenedione is the one that's kept it going. This adrenal hormone appears to be a far more potent stimulator of testosterone production than DHEA. The reason is simple. It takes the body two steps to convert DHEA to testosterone. Yet, it takes only one step for androstenedione. In fact, androstenedione is the intermediary step between DHEA and testosterone.

Use of this direct testosterone precursor as an anabolic agent was first tested by researchers in 1962. They gave a few women 100mg of androstenedione orally and measured their blood testosterone levels over a 90 minute period. They found that the supplement produced a 300% increase in blood testosterone in 60 minutes. In 90 minutes, levels were down to half of peak values. From this we see that androstenedione acts potently as a testosterone booster but also fades quickly.

German researchers looked into this compound in the early 1980's and even filed a patent application for use of androstenedione as an anabolic agent. One of the studies cited in the patent showed oral doses of 50 mg and 100 mg given to healthy men raised testosterone levels by 140% to 183% and 211% to 237% respectively. (9)

East German athletes and researchers caught wind of this research and began to perform some test of their own. They found that while oral ingestion did indeed increase testosterone, using it in a nasal spray was even more effective.

The idea of nasal application is intriguing and actually makes a lot of sense. A hormone substance like androstenedione is a somewhat fragile organic molecule. When it hits the acidic environment of the stomach, the molecule may be damaged and its activity diminished. However, it's also very well recognized by the body and easily absorbed through a porous membrane, like that in the nose. So, if snorted, it gets into the bloodstream without being exposed to the gut, thus maintaining its powerful biological activity.

Both DHEA and adrostenedione are direct precursors to testosterone and may increase production in the body simply by supplying more raw materials. Yet there are other ways to boost your body's natural testosterone production.

Tribulus Terrestris: Herbal Testosterone Booster

Originally introduced to support the sports supplement market by a small California based company under the brand name "Tribestan", this herbal extract, originating in Bulgaria, has become very popular in the bodybuilding world. It has been promoted as a testosterone booster from the beginning in the United States, but in Bulgaria, it has been used for years as a treatment for impotency and infertility. Although Tribulus Terrestris has been used as a treatment for decades, no one ever really understood why it worked - at least not until the early 1980's. It was then that researchers at the Chemical Pharmaceutical Research Institute in Sofia, Bulgaria began to study the biological effects of this potent herb.

Researchers found Tribulus Terrestris may have the ability to increase natural testosterone production by boosting levels of something called "luteinizing hormone" (LH), a pituitary hormone responsible for regulating testosterone levels. LH actually turns on natural testosterone production. One of the Research Institute's revealed that a daily dose of 750 mg of Tribulus Terrestris given to healthy mean increased their LH by an average of 72% and subsequently hiked free testosterone levels by an impressive 41%. (10)

So, far we've investigated two hormone substrates (DHEA and androstenedione) - raw materials for testosterone production - as well as a substance (Tribulus Terrestris) which may stimulate testosterone production. This natural testosterone producing stack is an extremely potent combination. But there is a way to make it even more effective.

The problem with the testosterone boosting power of combining DHEA, androstenedione and Tribulus Terrestris is that it is relatively short lived. Hormone levels appear to return to baseline levels within a few hours after taking a dose. The question is "how much does this quick testosterone boost increase muscle growth?" Are testosterone levels increased enough for a sufficient period of time to produce steroid like gains in muscle mass? The only honest answer to those questions is that nobody knows.

Anecdotal evidence from athletes currently using the stack suggests it probably does have some positive effects on performance / strength, and it may even boost muscle growth. A few athletes who are experimenting with this unique supplement stack, who have also tried steroids, commented that it produced mild steroid like effects.

So, just how much testosterone do you need to boost muscle growth? Well, it's probably not necessary to enhance serum testosterone levels by 300% or more to accelerate muscle growth. If moderate increases in testosterone (say 50% to 100%) could be achieved and maintained, the effects on muscle mass could be optimized - while concurrently decreasing the risk of possible undesirable effects.

Other questions which come up often are "how long should I take this stuff?" "Should I cycle it?" "If I decide to take three time the recommended dose, will I get three times the results?"

Typically, when you manipulate the biological balance of your body in any form - be it through chronic consumption of coffee, steroid use, or even extended use of such non-steroidal anti-inflammatory drugs like aspirin or ibuprofen - your body will fight back. It will react to what it perceives as an imbalance and try to set it straight.

It is well known that chronic use of anabolic steroids can lead to alterations in natural hormone production. This happens because the body perceives an unnatural increase in testosterone and the byproducts of testosterone. The system's natural response is to shut down the internal metabolic pathways of testosterone production to try and bring levels back into the normal range.

So, will use of natural testosterone enhancing nutrients lead to the same self-regulating effects? The answer is - maybe, maybe not.

Although the end results of steroid use and natural testosterone enhancement may be similar - albeit to different degrees - there are other key differences which are important to the way the body handles the situation. When huge doses of synthetic testosterone or testosterone derivatives (anabolic steroids) are introduced directly into the bloodstream, serum androgen levels skyrocket. Not only that, but these drugs are already in a biologically active form; thus, they bypass all of the steps in the normal metabolic pathway to testosterone production. By doing so, they completely overwhelm the system and over-ride all natural testosterone production activities, shutting them down quickly.

On the other hand, natural stimulation of testosterone production through the introduction of natural substrates and pro-hormones is different. These compounds are not yet in an active form, so they must be converted through enzymatic activity along the normal pathway of testosterone production to be activated. On top of that, by stimulating LH production, Tribulus Terrestris may drive the natural production of testosterone, thus continually activating the natural metabolic pathway.

The necessity of substrate conversion and natural pathway stimulation offers two possible helpful effects. First, it slows down the introduction of active testosterone into the system. This may help blunt the body's perception of imbalance and thus the equalizing actions typically seen with steroid use. Second, many of the enzymes and organs involved in normal testosterone production are kept active. This may help avoid inactivation and eventual dormancy of these systems as is seen with extended use of anabolic drugs.

What can be done, then, to allow these supplements to work better for longer? To answer that question we need to dig a little into the science of testosterone biochemistry.

There are two main responses by which the body attempts to deal with a perceived excess of serum testosterone. First, it up regulates the processes of testosterone clearance. It does so via two main pathways of testosterone degradation and clearance. One pathway leads to the formation of estrogen and the other to dihydrotestosterone (DHT). Not only does this increased clearance over time lead to less effect from supplementation, the end metabolites of these clearance pathways (namely, estrogen and DHT) happen to be responsible for most of the undesirable effects experienced by some long term steroid users. Excess estrogen accumulation can, for instance, cause water retention and even gynecomastia in serious cases. And elevated DHT level may lead to enlargement of the prostrate.

Another way the body tries to counteract excess testosterone accumulation is by slowing production of LH, which in turn slows down stimulation of testosterone production. The way it does this is closely connected to the increase in testosterone clearance mentioned above. The pituitary gland (which secretes LH) doesn't only gauge levels in the bloodstream, it regulates its LH producing activity. In actuality, the pituitary is highly sensitive to serum levels of estrogen. So, as testosterone levels build up in the blood, it's not only the testosterone causing the shutdown of LH secretion but also estrogen created secondary to increased conversion of testosterone through the estrogen clearance pathway. **To put it simply, increased estrogen production shuts down testosterone production!**

The combination of the two reactive mechanisms just described are quite effective for eventually bringing blood levels of testosterone back into what the body considers the normal range. The main culprit in this scenario is really the body's ability to increase the efficiency of testosterone clearance.

Obviously, enhanced testosterone clearance has its drawbacks. Not only will it more than likely end up suppressing natural LH and subsequent testosterone production, it may also create some undesirable effects. Decreasing or even halting the process of testosterone conversion to DHT and estrogen would obviously help attenuate these undesirable effects as well as extend the active half-life of testosterone in the system.

To achieve this goal, many steroid users rely on the use of more drugs - the most popular being Cytadren, Teslac and Nolvadex. These drugs are used as anti-estrogenic compounds. They exert their effects by blocking the formation of estrogen from testosterone through inactivation of the enzyme necessary to complete the conversion, or they block receptors for estrogen. For those of us who aren't interested in getting involved in prescription drug use, our options are limited

- but, exciting research shows that there **are** options.

The testosterone boosting stack as described is hugely powerful - offering the ability to increase natural testosterone production by 100%. Yet, for a product to be a true steroid alternative, it will have to have all of the following:

Potent testosterone enhancing effects

A delivery system which protects sensitive ingredients such as androstenedione and DHEA

A delivery which creates a slow, steady release of nutrients into the system, thus sustaining a more even and longer lasting testosterone enhancing effect.

The ability to minimize or halt conversion to both estrogen and DHT.

In recent years a number of companies have taken on the challenge of producing a testosterone booster that meets all four of these criteria. A few of them have succeeded. The first to do so was EAS, who released Andro-6 as their star testosterone boosting product. Others have followed. These products have been producing some pretty amazing results. Here's a run-down on how they work and why you need to get hold of them.

Firstly the ultimate T-stack must contain precise levels of each of the potent testosterone enhancers - androstenedione, DHEA and Tribulus Terrestris. On top of this, ensure that your stack of choice has an additional trio of natural compounds to the formula which, according to scientific studies, not only block conversion of testosterone to estrogen and DHT but also helps clear excess estrogen from the system as well. What are these 3 extra key players?

Saw Palmetto: The DHT Defender

Saw Palmetto is a potent herb derived from the berries of a small palm tree found in the South Eastern United States, and it has become quite popular in the field of complimentary health care. It is mainly used in the treatment of a condition known as benign prostatic hyperplasia (BHP), which is more commonly called enlargement of the prostate. When testosterone levels in the body increase, so does the rate of DHT formation. Scientists have discovered that it may be this conversion of testosterone to DHT in the prostate which causes prostate cells to multiply excessively, leading to prostate enlargement. Recently, researchers have discovered that saw palmetto extract may inhibit this conversion of testosterone to DHT, in addition to blocking the DHT receptor sites in the prostate.

This inhibition of DHT formation serves two very vital purposes. First, it helps guard against the possible increase in prostatic cellular growth. Secondly, by blocking the DHT conversion pathway of testosterone degradation, it may have the added benefit of

183

actually supporting higher levels and a longer half-life of active testosterone in the system. On top of all of this saw palmetto has also been shown to have possess anti-estrogenic effects.

Chrysin: A Natural Estrogen Enemy

Chrysin is a natural botanical nutrient that has potent anti-estrogenic effects. In one study it was shown to have almost identical anti-estrogenic activity as Cytadren (a popular anti-estrogenic steroid). The suppression of the conversion of testosterone to estrogen has far reaching ramifications related to natural testosterone enhancement. First, by decreasing estrogen production, pituitary LH secretion in maintained (or possibly even enhanced), thus supporting continued testosterone production. This mechanism is supported by anti-estrogenic drug research.

www.ingramcontent.com/pod-product-compliance
Lightning Source LLC
Chambersburg PA
CBHW060326030426
42336CB00011B/1228